The Resource Guide for the Disabled

The
Resource Guide
for the Disabled

Gayle Backstrom

TAYLOR PUBLISHING COMPANY
Dallas, Texas

*To Maurine Burnett, without whom I could not
have managed in coping with my own disability.*

Published by Taylor Publishing Company
        1550 West Mockingbird Lane
        Dallas, Texas 75235

Library of Congress Cataloging-in-Publication Data

Backstrom, Gayle.
    The resource guide for the disabled / Gayle Backstrom.
        p.   cm.
    Includes index.
    ISBN 0-87833-845-4
    1. Physically handicapped—Services for—United States—
Directories.   2. Chronically ill—Services for—United States—
Directories.   I. Title.
HV3023.A2B33   1994
362.4'048'02573—dc20   94–150
                                                         CIP

Printed in the United States of America

10   9   8   7   6   5   4   3   2   1

Acknowledgments

The research for this book has taken almost a full year, and I would not have been able to locate as many resources as I have without the help of the reference staff at the Denton Public Library, Linda Touraine, Carol Weller, and Marilyn Williams; the librarians at the Government Documents office at the University of North Texas Library, also in Denton, Texas; and Sandra Masten of the United Way in Denton. Lorena Jones, my editor, has been a constant source of assistance as we debated which material to include and how to organize it. I truly believe I am fortunate to have her as my editor.

CONTENTS

Introduction

When I wrote my first book, *When Muscle Pain Won't Go Away,* I wanted to include as many resources in it as possible and, incidentally, it was the list of resources that drew the most compliments when the book was published. I learned then that there is a lot of help available if you just know how to find it. Unfortunately, that is often the problem. Many people don't know where to go for help, regardless of the type of assistance they need.

About the time I started thinking about writing my second book, my sister, Phyllis, was declared legally blind and fighting depression. And my other sister, Shirley, was trying to help her son cope with juvenile diabetes—without much success. I knew we could find helpful sources if we just looked hard enough and, thus, the idea for *The Resource Guide for the Disabled* was born.

I have spent almost a year working on this book, but I know I could spend another one, or two, or even more accumulating resources. However, that book would be so expensive it would defeat the purpose. My editor and I agreed that this book would be for the average individual—not like the huge volumes that social workers and other service providers rely on.

I have included about 500 resources here that I believe will give those with disabilities or chronic illnesses a good start on finding help. These sources range from groups such as Emotions Anonymous to Wheelchair Aviators and the Small Business Administration's Handicap Loan Program. I have listed many governmental programs, including those that offer a range of services from providing educational grants and medical care to funding the latest research on cancer, arthritis, spinal cord injuries, and other serious health problems. You will find that governmental programs also provide information and assistance to help carry out the new Americans with Disabilities Act.

Although the number of actual resources listed here is approximately 500, these 500 should be multiplied by the number of state, regional, or local offices as well as specific local chapters. The total number of contacts lies somewhere in the thousands. No matter what information you are looking for or what assistance you need, there is almost always someone available who can help within one or two phone calls. I wish you the best as you reach out for a resource.

How to Use this Book

A brief explanation of how to read the entries, along with a couple of general guidelines to keep in mind, will help you get the most out of the resources that follow. Here's what you need to know to put this book to work for you.

Sometimes a resource may offer additional services, but I have included only those that I found to be available as I gathered my information. Some resources are strictly local, but are included because they are good models and, in many cases, are willing to share information with others interested in starting similar programs in another area.

Not all of the services are available directly to individuals or their families. Some programs work through state agencies, such as the vocational rehabilitation offices. (The programs are funded and mandated by the federal government, but each state has set up its own vocational rehabilitation program with regional and local offices.) Some programs are set up through the local school district. (Hence, every child is guaranteed an education regardless of his or her physical or mental status.) Although you cannot deal directly with these kinds of resources, understanding their function and services can help you benefit through another party.

Here is a breakdown of the format I have set up for the entries, explaining what kind of organization a resource is, who it helps, and what their services are as well as which disability or chronic illness it serves:

Organization name

While this should be a simple matter, it isn't always. Many governmental programs are listed under a particular department and then under a division within that department. Whenever possible, that information immediately follows the department name or appears within the comments. One example is the U.S. Department of Education. There are several divisions within this department, such as Special Education and Rehabilitation and Secondary Education. Within those divisions, the various programs are then named.

Contact name

Only a few individual names are listed to allow for the inevitable changes in personnel. The names that are listed are either those who are resources themselves or who are so closely linked to the resource that they cannot be discounted.

Address

Again, this is generally self-explanatory, although many of the governmental programs' addresses do not have an actual street or post office box address.

Telephone and fax number

The first phone number listed is an 800 number if the organization has one. Sometimes the 800 number is restricted to those within one state or in all but one state. (Such restrictions are noted.) If an 800 number is not offered, the organization's main number is listed first. An alternate number, if it exists, is listed second. If there is a number for the Telecommunications Device for the Deaf (TDD), it is indicated. (Some organizations have a separate number for these special communications for the deaf or hard of hearing, but some have numbers that offer both voice and TDD.) Whenever possible, I have listed a fax number. Some of the governmental offices use the same number for both voice and fax.

Type of organization

Be aware that some organizations are not categorized as strictly one type—combinations do exist here. For example, there are private, non-profit agencies and colleges or universities that are also medical and/or research facilities.

Public served

Generally, a resource can and will serve more than one public. Any of the national organizations for various health conditions, such as the Arthritis Foundation and the American Cancer Society, will provide information to individuals and family members but will also respond to the general public, media, and medical community. Many of these organizations have medical professionals on their boards or committees, and they almost always support research.

Other organizations may serve only the medical community, researchers, or nonmedical professionals, just as many other programs deal only with intermediate parties. An example of the latter is a HUD housing loan or rental assistance program that goes to an intermediate party, such as a public housing project or local financial institution, who then facilitates the dispersal of funds. Please understand these stipulations and use such information properly; a national office will direct you to an intermediate party, but it cannot help you directly.

Offers

Almost all of the resources can give you information. This may include the contact name and phone number at the local or regional office, a complete packet of brochures, bibliographies, and more. Some organizations offer a wide range of services and some provide only one. This does not mean that it isn't worthwhile to check out that one service. For example, many of the recreational services open the door to a world of sports participation opportunities, which then leads individuals to social activities, increased self-esteem, and much more.

Sometimes it is difficult to describe what an organization or agency provides in one word. A good example is the guide dog programs. Is a guide dog a product or a living aid? To prevent confusion, I classified it as both and offered further explanation in the comments.

You will find relevant professional organizations among the listings. Some of them may give local referrals and others may not—there is no general rule. I have included them because often they give individuals their guidelines, which explain how members and officers are selected.

Many times, I included only a portion of the information on an organization's activities; you will have to go to that organization for more extensive information. When doing so, please be patient and consider the budgetary limitations many of these resources face. In these tough economic times, nonprofit organizations have had to cope with decreased donations and cutbacks in governmental funding on every level. Also keep in mind that in the effort to balance the budget, it is likely that some of the governmental programs listed may be cut entirely or severely downscaled.

Regardless of funding difficulties, I always found staff members and volunteers eager to provide information about their organization, even though the one person in the office was quite busy (often there is only a one- or two-person staff). When you request information, ask when you can expect a response and accept that schedule. After all, they are there to provide services but no one is a miracle worker; they often face limitations of one sort or another.

Most of the time the information is free, although there may be a charge for some of the publications. **Not every resource offers free assistance.** This book is not just a listing of free help. In certain cases, a client's fees will be adjusted because of their financial status, but always ask about charges.

Disability/chronic illness

When I began to gather information, I thought this section would be very cut and dry. But, as the resources accumulated, I found it wasn't always that simple. Some programs, such as Pell Grants and Guaranteed Student Loans, are available to anyone, including able-bodied individuals. I have listed such programs because eligibility is often based on financial need and many people with disabilities or chronic illnesses fall squarely into that category. Anytime I found such a program or one that was open to those with any disability or chronic illness, I simply noted "All." Other organizations help anyone who has multiple handicaps (such as mental retardation and blindness) or who has a mobility problem. And some organizations, such as the Epilepsy Foundation or Neurotics Anonymous, strictly work with those who have a specific disability or chronic illness.

Comments

This section includes everything from special information about telephone numbers to mission statements. Here I have noted when a nationwide organization has local chapters.

Where to Go from Here

As I explained in the Introduction, there is no way one book can list all the available resources. On a national or regional level there are at least another thousand in addition to the ones I found during my research, and that doesn't include the ones on the local level, which also climbs into the thousands. But how do you find those resources? Where do you turn for information on those local orgnizations?

Many places will lead you to additional resources. Almost every midsized town has a United Way office. Basically, the United Way raises funds and distributes them to various programs in the community. They also act as an information and referral office. While researching, I was told that every county is supposed to have an information and referral office where individuals can go to learn about the assistance that the community offers. However, not every county or town actually has such an office. If your community is one of those that does not, where do you go for help? The United Way office. The United Way often serves as a local information and referral office.

If you do not have access to a local information and referral office or a United Way office, you can start your search a couple of other places. Try the chamber of commerce, county judge's office, various city offices, or local ministerial alliance. Of course, many cities and counties have human services departments that provide assistance through food stamps, welfare, and aid to those with dependent children. Some larger cities have an office that deals strictly with the needs of those with disabilities.

I have lived in small towns as well as suburbs of large metropolitan areas. Even in the smallest town, the local church officials have usually formed a ministerial alliance. Sometimes the alliance is informal and primarily exists to decide who will preside at the combined holiday services. Other alliances have coordinated their giving programs so that those in need may go directly to that office rather than going from one church to another seeking assistance. The assistance may be come from a "clothes closet," which offers good quality used clothing for free or a nominal charge, or a food bank. In larger communities, the churches may pass on funds designated for the needy to a central office and the assistance takes the form of helping individuals pay for their utilities or housing in emergency cases. Many churches and synagogues also offer counseling services. (In smaller communities, one or two of the local ministers or rabbis will have had specialized counseling training.) More established organizations, such as the Lutheran Family Services or Catholic Charities, will commonly have a office in larger cities.

Check with the county and city to reach their department of human services, housing, or public health office. Many services are available on a sliding scale or for free, but eligibilty requirements vary according to the amount of money available so be sure to ask. Most cities also have a parks and recreation department that offers free or low-cost activities ranging from sports to arts, which often includes programs specially designed for the disabled.

You can also check with the social workers at the local public hospital. Almost every hospital has at least one social worker on staff or on retainer who can give you the names and contacts for programs that might help you. Contrary to common belief, you do not have to be a patient (or past patient) at the hospital for the social workers to assist you. Also be aware that many hospitals provide meeting space for support groups.

Of course, the local library can be a source of local as well as national resources. Quite often reference librarians are especially knowledgeable about the resources in their county. If none of the resources they recommend meets your needs, the librarian can help you find the phone numbers and addresses for national and regional resources. The *Encyclopedia of Associations* is another excellent source that is updated annually. There are also countless books written specifically for particular disabilities and chronic illnesses; check them for resource information.

Local school districts also provide many services. Most of them are covered in the governmental listings under the U.S. Department of

Education, but additional services that are more localized may exist. Check also with the Regional Education Service Center. If you don't know where the closest one is, call the local superintendent's office.

Investigate any recreational opportunities at the local boys' and girls' clubs, YMCA and YWCA, and Camp Fire associations. Many local civic groups sponsor programs for the handicapped. If you don't know anyone in the Lion's Club, Rotary, Junior League, Jaycees or other similar organization, call the chamber of commerce or local newspaper for the president's name and phone number.

Other sources of help, such as a county agricultural extension agent or Consumer Credit Counseling, may be more specialized but indirectly related to a disability or chronic illness. For example, an extension agent might be able to provide information on nutrition and Consumer Credit Counseling (a nonprofit organization that helps individuals and families with financial matters) could help an individual work with creditors in an emergency situation.

The nearest college or university can be another major resource. Services offered are dependent on the existing college degree programs and can include assistance in dental hygiene, physical therapy, occupational therapy, family counseling, and speech and language therapy. If a medical school exists, medical services may be available at reduced rates. Typically, universities have research programs that use volunteers in their studies. Although volunteers are not generally paid, the medical services are usually free and a minor reimbursement for travel expenses may be provided. Some universities also have a center for rehabilitation studies where, individuals are evaluated and given rehabilitative services. Costs will vary.

As you can see, a wide variety of help is available once you begin to look for it. It is not all free, nor is it all financially related, but when you need help be sure to consider all that is available. Although you may think that what you really need is an extra $250 (or $500 or whatever) a month, you may be able to go to Consumer Credit Counseling and learn how to better manage what you do have. You may be able to get into a university health science center or clinic at a reduced rate. Or, you might find a recreational program for your developmentally disabled child that will not only bring him or her pleasure but that will also give you a break from childcare.

Start by sitting down and determining just what help you need. Look through this book to find any resources that could help, contact them, and ask for more referrals. Amazingly, each resource always leads to others. Keep a record of who you contact and what, specifically, their response was so you don't repeat your efforts and waste time.

Again, I wish you the best in your search and pray that the assistance you receive will make your disability or chronic illness a little easier to bear. Good luck and let me hear from you.

A

52 ASSOCIATION FOR THE HANDICAPPED
350 Fifth Ave., Ste. 1829
New York, NY 10118
212–563–9797
FAX: 212–563–2693

Type of organization: nonprofit
Public served: individuals/families
Offers: information, recreational
   opportunities
Disability/chronic illness: physical
   disabilities, including amputation and blindness (in veterans)

Comments: Provides 8,000 veterans who are amputees, paraple-
gics, or blind, as well as similarly
handicapped civilians, with Confidence Through Sports programs
at its outdoor sports and recreation center in Ossining, NY.
Conducts ski clinics for amputees
and the blind at ski areas in the
U.S. during winter months.

ABLEDATA, NATIONAL REHABILITATION INFORMATION CENTER
8455 Colesville Rd., Ste. 935
Silver Spring, MD 20910
1–800–346–2742
301–588–9284

Type of organization: private
Public served: individuals/families,
   general public, media, medical
   personnel
Offers: information, consulta-
   tions/guidance, products,
   rehabilitative services
Disability/chronic illness: all

Comments: Provides information
on commercially available rehabilitation and independent-living
equipment for persons with disabilities.

ACCENT ON LIVING (and Accent Special Publications)
P.O. Box 700
Bloomington, IL 61702
309–378–2961

Type of organization: private
Public served: individuals/families,
   general public, media, medical
   personnel
Offers: information, publica-
   tion(s)
Disability/chronic illness: all

Comments: *Accent on Living* is a
quarterly magazine with information for those with all types of
physical disabilities; mostly for
adults. Accent Special Publications publishes and sells books
dealing with disabilities. Write for
their free catalog.

1

ACCESS TO RECREATION

2509 East Thousand Oaks Blvd.,
    Ste. 430
Thousand Oaks, CA 91362
1–800–634–4351
805–498–7535

Type of organization: private
Public served: individuals/families,
    general public
Offers: recreational opportunities,
    products, living aids
Disability/chronic illness: all

Comments: Provides a catalog of
adaptive recreational equipment
and living aids for the elderly and
disabled.

ACCESS USA NEWS

Roadrunner Publishing Inc.
P.O. Box 1134
Crystal Lake, IL 60039
815–363–0900
815–363–0922 (TDD)
FAX: 815–363–0923

Type of organization: private
Public served: individuals/families,
    general public, media, medical
    personnel, nonmedical profes-
    sionals
Offers: information, publica-
    tion(s)
Disability/chronic illness: all

Comments: A lifestyle magazine
for people with disabilities.

ACF TECHNOLOGY, INC.

1400 Lee Dr., Ste. 3
Coraopolis, PA 15108
412–264–2288
FAX: 412–269–6675

Type of organization: private
Public served: individuals/families,
    general public
Offers: products
Disability/chronic illness: speech
    handicaps

Comments: Offers speech pros-
theses.

A CHANCE TO GROW

3820 Emerson Ave. North
Minneapolis, MN 55412
612–521–2266
FAX: 612–521–9647

Type of organization: nonprofit
Public served: individuals/families,
    general public, media
Offers: information, education,
    diagnostic services, reference
    material, publication(s), sup-
    port group(s), nonmedical
    referrals, consultations/guid-
    ance, seminars/workshops,
    rehabilitative services, voca-
    tional services
Disability/chronic illness: head
    injury

Comments: Offers a wide variety
of services, most involved with

2

brain injuries and relearning. Includes brain rehabilitation, by therapy as a physical intervention process to rebuild the brain, and biofeedback training for attention deficit and hyperactive children. Operates a home health agency and day school for those with learning or visual perception problems.

ACHILLES TRACK CLUB
1 Times Square, 10th Fl.
New York, NY 10036
212–354–0300
FAX: 212–354–3978

Type of organization: nonprofit
Public served: individuals/families
Offers: information, support
   group(s), recreational
   opportunities
Disability/chronic illness: all

Comments: Has 40 local groups with international members interacting by mail. Members include disabled runners and volunteer coaches. Purpose is to encourage people with all types of disabilities to participate in running, and to improve the self-image of the disabled and demonstrate that they are energetic and capable people. Encourages the disabled to be aerobically fit and to run in competitions beside the able-bodied.

ACTION, FOSTER GRANDPARENT PROGRAM
1100 Vermont Ave. NW
Washington, DC 20525
202–606–4851

Type of organization: government
Public served: individuals/families,
   intermediate parties
Offers: education, supportive
   services
Disability/chronic illness: all

Comments: Foster grandparents work with infants, children, or youth who have special needs because of physical, mental, or emotional problems. Generally, work is done at residential and nonresidential facilities, including preschool establishments, schools, and homes. Foster grandparents are low-income persons age 60 and older. Call national office in Washington for information on the nearest program.

ACTION, SENIOR COMPANION GRANDPARENT PROGRAM
1100 Vermont Ave. NW
Washington, DC 20525
202–606–4851

Type of organization: government
Public served: individuals/families,
   intermediate parties

Offers: supportive services
Disability/chronic illness: all

Comments: Senior Companion Grandparent Program works to provide volunteer opportunities for low-income persons 60 or older that enhance their ability to remain active and provide critically needed community services. Primarily helps older people with mental, emotional, and physical impairments achieve and maintain their fullest health potential and manage their lives independently.

ADAPTABILITY
Mill Street
Colchester, CT 06415
1–800–243–9232
203–537–3451

Type of organization: private
Public served: individuals/families
Offers: products
Disability/chronic illness: physical disabilities

Comments: Source for daily living aids; offers free catalog.

ADVANCED MOBILITY SYSTEMS OF TEXAS
2105 A Beach St.
Fort Worth, TX 76111
817–834–1003

Type of organization: private
Public served: individuals/families
Offers: products
Disability/chronic illness: physical disabilities

Comments: Source for van conversions, lifts, wheelchairs, medical supplies.

ADVENTURES IN MOVEMENT FOR THE HANDICAPPED
945 Danbury Rd.
Dayton, OH 45420
1–800–332–8210
513–294–4611
FAX: 513–294–3783

Type of organization: nonprofit
Public served: individuals/families, nonmedical professionals
Offers: recreational opportunties
Disability/chronic illness: all

Comments: Has developed movement training and swimming programs that are exclusively for children.

ADVOCACY CENTER FOR THE ELDERLY AND DISABLED
210 O'Keefe Ave., Ste. 700
New Orleans, LA 70112
1–800–960–7705 (in LA)
504–522–2337
FAX: 504–522–5507

4

Type of organization: nonprofit, private
Public served: individuals/families
Offers: information, civil rights assistance/advocacy
Disability/chronic illness: developmental disabilities, geriatric disabilities and physical/mental illnesses

Comments: Interested in sociolegal problems; provides general reference services, and conducts seminars. Serves clients of Louisiana Rehabilitation Services and nursing homes; services free to elderly citizens of parishes under contract with Councils on Aging.

AFFILIATED LEADERSHIP LEAGUE OF AND FOR THE BLIND OF AMERICA
1101 17th St. NW, #803
Washington, DC 20036
202–833–0092
FAX: 202–833–0086

Type of organization: nonprofit, private
Public served: intermediate parties
Offers: consultations/guidance, civil rights assistance/advocacy
Disability/chronic illness: visual impairments

Comments: Involved in policy development on blindness issues for various service organizations.

AIDS AND SEXUALLY TRANSMITTED DISEASES RESOURCE CENTER
1–800–227–8922

Type of organization: nonprofit
Public served: individuals/families, general public
Offers: information, medical referrals
Disability/chronic illness: AIDS and sexually transmitted diseases

Comments: Operates 8 A.M. to 8 P.M., Pacific Standard Time. Provides referrals to clinics and support groups and other services. Offers brochures and pamphlets.

AIDS HOTLINE
1–800–342–2437
1–800–243–7889 (TDD)

Type of organization: private
Public served: individuals/families, general public, media
Offers: information, publication(s), medical referrals, nonmedical referrals
Disability/chronic illness: AIDS

Comments: Call 1–800–342–7432 for information in Spanish. Can also provide national referrals.

ALABAMA DEPARTMENT OF EDUCATION, REFERRAL FOR DISABLED CHILDREN
Montgomery, AL
1–800–543–3098 (in AL)
205–242–9950

Type of organization: government
Public served: individuals/families
Offers: information, education
Disability/chronic illness: all

Comments: For Alabama children only.

ALEXANDER GRAHAM BELL ASSOCIATION FOR THE DEAF
3417 Volta Pl. NW
Washington, DC 20007
202–337–5220 (voice and TDD)

Type of organization: nonprofit
Public served: individuals/families, general public, media
Offers: information, seminars/ workshops, financial assistance
Disability/chronic illness: hearing impairments

Comments: Offers college scholarships for the hearing impaired.

ALFRED I. DUPONT INSTITUTE, MEDICAL LIBRARY
P.O. Box 269
Wilmington, DE 19899
302–651–5820

Type of organization: private, medical facility
Public served: individuals/families, general public, media, medical personnel
Offers: information, diagnostic services, reference material, medical referrals, medical services, consultations/guidance, seminars/workshops, research material
Disability/chronic illness: all

Comments: Medical facility is a multispecialty children's hospital.

ALZHEIMER'S ASSOCIATION, NATIONAL HEADQUARTERS
919 North Michigan Ave.,
Ste. 1000
Chicago, IL 60611–1676
1–800–272–3900
312–335–8700
FAX: 312–335–1110

Type of organization: nonprofit
Public served: individuals/families, general public, media, medical personnel, nonmedical professionals
Offers: information, nonmedical referrals, seminars/workshops
Disability/chronic illness: Alzheimer's disease

Comments: Has more than 223 local chapters. Services vary from one chapter to another; depending on fundraising, some have workshops for nursing home and other professionals. Contact local chapter for support groups and counseling.

AMC CANCER RESEARCH CENTER AND HOSPITAL MEDICAL LIBRARY
1600 Pierce St.
Denver, CO 80214
1-800-525-3777*
303-233-6501

Type of organization: private, medical, research facility
Public served: individuals/families, general public, media, medical personnel, researchers
Offers: information, reference material, publication(s), medical referrals, research material
Disability/chronic illness: cancer

Comments: *In the U.S., except CO.

AMERICAN ACADEMY FOR CEREBRAL PALSY AND DEVELOPMENTAL MEDICINE
P.O. Box 11086
Richmond, VA 23230
804-282-0036
FAX: 804-282-0090

Type of organization: professional
Public served: medical personnel
Offers: information

Disability/chronic illness: cerebral palsy and developmental disabilities (in children)

Comments: A professional organization; has recommended reading list for parents.

AMERICAN ACADEMY OF FACIAL, PLASTIC & RECONSTRUCTIVE SURGERY
1101 Vermont Ave. NW
Washington, DC 20005
1-800-332-3223
202-842-4500
FAX: 202-371-1514

Type of organization: professional
Public served: individuals/families, general public, media, medical personnel
Offers: information, medical referrals
Disability/chronic illness: severe burns and craniofacial deformities

Comments: A professional association.

AMERICAN ALLIANCE FOR HEALTH, PHYSICAL EDUCATION, RECREATION AND DANCE
1900 Association Dr.
Reston, VA 22091
1-800-321-0789*
703-476-3400
FAX: 703-476-9527

Type of organization: professional
Public served: individuals/families, nonmedical professionals
Offers: information, publication(s), recreational opportunities
Disability/chronic illness: all

Comments: *For book orders only. Alliance consists of associations involved in the four areas.

AMERICAN AMPUTEE FOUNDATION
Box 250218
Little Rock, AR 72225
501–666–2523
FAX: 501–666–8367

Type of organization: nonprofit
Public served: individuals/families
Offers: information, reference material, publication(s), support group(s), counseling, nonmedical referrals, seminars/workshops, financial assistance, civil rights assistance/advocacy, products, rehabilitative services
Disability/chronic illness: amputation, some spinal cord injuries if no other help is available

Comments: Offers peer counseling to help new amputees adjust, as well as information and referrals, legal assistance, technical and scientific information on prosthetics, and financial aid for prosthetic equipment, wheelchairs, crutches, braces, modifications to the home, and more.

AMERICAN ASSOCIATION FOR THE ADVANCEMENT OF SCIENCE, PROJECT ON THE HANDICAPPED IN SCIENCE
1333 H St. NW
Washington, DC 20005
202–326–6400
FAX: 202–371–9849

Type of organization: professional
Public served: individuals/families, nonmedical professionals
Offers: information, publication(s), counseling, vocational services
Disability/chronic illness: physical, visual, hearing, learning, or speech impairments

Comments: The association promotes the disabled's entry into the fields of science, math, and engineering by providing mentors. *The Resource Directory of Scientists and Engineers with Disabilities* provides professional contacts for young and midcareer scientists and engineers with disabilities.

AMERICAN ASSOCIATION OF RETIRED PERSONS (AARP)
601 East St. NW
Washington, DC 20049
202–434–2300
202–434–2277

Type of organization: nonprofit
Public served: individuals/families, general public, media
Offers: information, publication(s)
Disability/chronic illness: all (in the elderly)

Comments: Has local chapters. To qualify for AARP membership, individuals must be 50 years of age or older.

AMERICAN ASSOCIATION OF UNIVERSITY AFFILIATED PROGRAMS FOR PERSONS WITH DEVELOPMENTAL DISABILITIES
8630 Fenton St., #410
Silver Spring, MD 20910
301–588–8252
301–588–3319 (TDD)
FAX: 301–588–2842

Type of organization: nonprofit
Public served: intermediate parties
Offers: civil rights assistance/advocacy
Disability/chronic illness: developmental disabilities

Comments: Only function is to lobby for rights of those with developmental disabilities.

AMERICAN ASSOCIATION ON MENTAL RETARDATION
1719 Kalorama Rd. NW
Washington, DC 20009
1–800–424–3688
202–387–1968

Type of organization: nonprofit
Public served: individuals/families, general public
Offers: information, publication(s), seminars/workshops
Disability/chronic illness: mental retardation

Comments: This is a membership organization.

AMERICAN ATHLETIC ASSOCIATION FOR THE DEAF
3607 Washington Blvd., No. 4
Ogden, UT 84403–1737
801–393–7916
FAX: 801–393–2263

Type of organization: nonprofit
Public served: individuals/families, general public, media
Offers: information, recreational opportunities
Disability/chronic illness: hearing impairments

9

Comments: Fosters athletic competition among the deaf; has 200 local groups. Sponsors competitions at state, regional, and national levels in basketball and softball, as well as participation in Comite International des Sports Silencieux, and World Games for Deaf.

AMERICAN BAR ASSOCIATION, COMMITTEE ON MENTAL AND PHYSICAL DISABLED LAW

1800 M St. NW
Washington, DC 20036
202-331-2240
FAX: 202-331-2220

Type of organization: professional organization
Public served: individuals/families, general public, media, non-medical professionals, intermediate parties
Offers: information, publication(s), civil rights assistance/advocacy
Disability/chronic illness: physical disabilities, mental retardation, developmental disabilities

Comments: The American Bar Association publishes *The Journal of Mental and Physical Disability Reporter,* which reviews cases concerning the ADA, six times a year. The association also provides referrals to protection and advocacy groups or to the bar association's Center for Children and the Law if children are involved.

AMERICAN BLIND BOWLING ASSOCIATION, INC.

c/o Alice M. Hoover
411 Sheriff St.
Mercer, PA 16137
412-662-5748

Type of organization: nonprofit
Public served: individuals/families
Offers: recreational opportunities
Disability/chronic illness: visual impairments

Comments: Has 140 local groups, open to men and women 18 and older who are legally blind. Holds tenpin bowling competitions and supports bowling as recreation.

AMERICAN BLIND SKIING FOUNDATION

610 South William St.
Mt. Prospect, IL 60056
708-255-1739

Type of organization: nonprofit
Public served: individuals/families
Offers: recreational opportunities
Disability/chronic illness: visual impairments

Comments: An organization of volunteers who teach downhill and cross-country recreational and competitive skiing to the blind and visually handicapped. Holds giant slalom, downhill, and cross-country races. Travels with blind skiers to skiing areas in Colorado, Wisconsin, and Michigan. Sponsors international races in Canada, the World Cup for the Disabled in Switzerland, and the Olympics for the Disabled in Austria.

AMERICAN CAMPING ASSOCIATION
5000 State Road 67 North
Martinsville, IN 46151
317–342–8456
FAX: 317–342–2065

Type of organization: nonprofit
Public served: individuals/families, general public
Offers: recreation
Disability/chronic illness: all children

Comments: Publishes a directory of camps for children, including those for disabled children.

AMERICAN CANCER SOCIETY
1599 Clifton Rd. NE
Atlanta, GA 30329
404–320–3333
FAX: 404–325–0230

Type of organization: nonprofit
Public served: individuals/families, general public, media, medical personnel
Offers: information, support group(s), counseling, medical referrals, seminars/workshops, research material
Disability/chronic illness: cancer

Comments: Has 58 divisions and approximately 3,000 units nationwide. Purpose is to provide research, education, and service for cancer patients. Many services offered, such as loan of medical equipment, transportation to medical appointments, and support groups.

AMERICAN CHRONIC PAIN ASSOCIATION
P.O. Box 850
Rocklin, CA 95677
916–632–0922
FAX: 916–632–3208

Type of organization: nonprofit
Public served: individuals/families, general public, media
Offers: information, publication(s), support group(s), nonmedical referrals, seminars/workshops
Disability/chronic illness: chronic pain

Comments: Has about 750 local chapters. Call national headquarters for chapters and information on "The Writing Connection," which is for those who want to correspond with others who have chronic pain.

AMERICAN CLEFT PALATE ASSOCIATION, UNIVERSITY OF PITTSBURGH

1218 Grandview Ave.
Pittsburgh, PA 15211
1-800-242-5338
1-800-23CLEFT(in PA)

Type of organization: college
Public served: individuals/families, general public, media
Offers: information, medical referrals
Disability/chronic illness: cleft palate

AMERICAN COLLEGE OF ALLERGY & IMMUNOLOGY

800 E. Northwest Highway, Ste. 1080
Palatine, IL 60067-6520
708-427-1200

Type of organization: professional
Public served: individuals/families, general public, medical personnel
Offers: medical referrals
Disability/chronic illness: asthma, allergies and immunological diseases

AMERICAN COLLEGE OF CARDIOLOGY

9111 Old Georgetown Rd.
Bethesda, MD 20814-1699
301-897-5400
FAX: 301-897-9745

Type of organization: professional
Public served: individuals/families, general public, media, medical personnel
Offers: medical referrals
Disability/chronic illness: cardio-vascular disease

AMERICAN COLLEGE OF RHEUMATOLOGY

60 Executive Park Dr. South, Ste. 150
Atlanta, GA 30329
404-633-3777
FAX: 404-633-1870

Type of organization: professional
Public served: individuals/families, general public, media, medical personnel
Offers: information, medical referrals
Disability/chronic illness: arthritis, musculoskeletal disorders

AMERICAN COUNCIL OF THE BLIND

1155 15th St. NW, Ste. 720
Washington, DC 20005
1–800–424–8666*
202–467–5081

Type of organization: nonprofit
Public served: individuals/families, general public, media
Offers: information, medical referrals, financial assistance, rehabilitative services, vocational services
Disability/chronic illness: visual impairments

Comments: *Information line; staff members are available at this number between 3 P.M. and 5:30 P.M. EST, Monday through Friday. To reach the Washington Connection, an information and education hotline, call the number between 6 P.M. and midnight on weeknights and weekends. Provides some college scholarships, advisory and referral services, some seminars, and will provide referrals to other sources in response to inquiries.

AMERICAN DEAF VOLLEYBALL ASSOCIATION

c/o Farley Warshaw
300 Roxborough St.
Rochester, NY 14619
716–475–6838

Type of organization: nonprofit
Public served: individuals/families
Offers: information, seminars/ workshops, recreational opportunities
Disability/chronic illness: hearing impairments

Comments: Has 86 amateur volleyball organizations nationwide. Seeks to provide volleyball camps, developmental programs, training, and workshops for hearing-impaired children and adults. Sponsors U.S. women's and men's volleyball teams in international sports competitions.

AMERICAN DIABETES ASSOCIATION

1660 Duke St.
Alexandria, VA 22314
1–800–232–3472*
703–549–1500

Type of organization: nonprofit
Public served: individuals/families, general public, media, researchers
Offers: information, publications(s), counseling, seminars/ workshops, research material
Disability/chronic illness: diabetes and its complications

Comments: *Check your local phone directory for local 800 numbers. Purpose is to promote a search for a cure for or prevention of diabetes and improve the health and well-being of those with diabetes and their families. Implements a four-point program for diabetes control, which includes patient, public, and professional education and supporting diabetes research. Has 600 affiliates in all 50 states.

AMERICAN DISABILITY ASSOCIATION

2121 8th Ave. North, Ste. 1623
Birmingham, AL 35203
205-323-3030
FAX: 205-520-0603

Type of organization: nonprofit
Public served: individuals/families
Offers: information, reference material, publication(s), support group(s), counseling
Disability/chronic illness: all

Comments: Support group for those with disabilities, maintains library and database on disability issues. Provides children's services, educational and research programs, and charitable services. Database, publication on-line, and electronic mail can be accessed by calling the central network hub at 205-854-9074 or 205-854-5863.

AMERICAN FOUNDATION FOR THE BLIND

15 West 16th St.
New York, NY 10011
1-800-232-5463
212-620-2000
FAX: 212-727-1279

Type of organization: nonprofit
Public served: individuals/families, general public, media, non-medical professionals
Offers: information, education, reference material, publication(s), medical referrals, nonmedical referrals, consultations/guidance, civil rights assistance/advocacy, research material, products, living aids, rehabilitative services, vocational services
Disability/chronic illness: visual impairments

Comments: 212-620-2147 is a hotline in New York. Foundation ensures the development, maintenance, and improvement of services for blind and visually impaired. Services range from recording and manufacturing of Talking Books (in conjunction with the Library of Congress) to maintaining a reference library and adapting, evaluating, manufacturing, and selling special devices and consumer products to help the blind and visually impaired live and work independently.

AMERICAN HEARING RESEARCH FOUNDATION

55 East Washington St.,
Ste. 2022
Chicago, IL 60602
312–726–9670

Type of organization: nonprofit
Public served: individuals/families, general public, media, medical personnel, researchers
Offers: information, publication(s), medical referrals, research material
Disability/chronic illness: hearing impairments

AMERICAN HEART ASSOCIATION

7272 Greenville Ave.
Dallas, TX 75231
214–373–6300
FAX: 214–706–1341

Type of organization: nonprofit
Public served: individuals/families, general public, media
Offers: information, support group(s), medical referrals, research material
Disability/chronic illness: cardiovascular disease

Comments: Has local chapters nationwide.

AMERICAN HORTICULTURAL THERAPY ASSOCIATION

362A Christopher Ave.
Gaithersburg, MD 20879
1–800–634–1603
301–948–3010
FAX: 301–869–2397

Type of organization: nonprofit
Public served: individuals/families
Offers: information, publication(s), recreational opportunities
Disability/chronic illness: all

Comments: Contact the association for information on horticultural therapy programs held throughout the U.S. Such programs are sponsored by a wide variety of organizations, ranging from rehabilitation facilities to community colleges and arboretums.

AMERICAN INSTITUTE FOR CANCER RESEARCH

500 North Washington St.
Falls Church, VA 22046
1–800–843–8114
703–237–0159

Type of organization: nonprofit
Public served: individuals/families, general public, researchers
Offers: information
Disability/chronic illness: cancer

Comments: Focuses on prevention and early signs, alerts public to unethical practioners and groups, supports cancer research, and conducts seminars.

AMERICAN INSTITUTE OF ARCHITECTS

1735 New York Ave. NW
Washington, DC 20006
1–800–365–ARCH
202–626–7310
FAX: 202–626–7587

Type of organization: professional
Public served: individuals/families, general public, intermediate parties
Offers: information, publication(s)
Disability/chronic illness: physical disabilities

Comments: Bibliographies available for literature on barrier-free designs up through 1991–1992, which are sold to the general public for $5. Now, they do custom searches for designs at $75 per hour plus expenses.

AMERICAN KIDNEY FUND

6110 Executive Blvd.,
  Ste. 1010
Rockville, MD 20852
1–800–638–8299
301–881–3052
FAX: 301–881–0898

Type of organization: nonprofit
Public served: individuals/families, medical personnel, researchers
Offers: information, financial assistance, research material
Disability/chronic illness: kidney disease

Comments: Assists in paying kidney patients' medical costs, promotes research through grants, and participates in organ donation and community service.

AMERICAN LIVER FOUNDATION

1425 Pompton Ave.
Cedar Grove, NJ 07009
1–800–223–0179
201–256–2550
FAX: 201–256–3214

Type of organization: nonprofit
Public served: individuals/families, general public, media, medical personnel, researchers
Offers: information, publication(s), medical referrals, seminars/workshops, research material
Disability/chronic illness: liver disease

Comments: Funds research and works to inform public about liver disease.

AMERICAN LUNG ASSOCIATION

1740 Broadway
New York, NY 10019–4374
1–800–LUNGUSA*
212–315–8700
FAX: 212–265–5642

Type of organization: nonprofit
Public served: individuals/families, general public, media, medical personnel
Offers: information, publication(s), support group(s), medical referrals, seminars/workshops
Disability/chronic illness: lung disease, cancer, emphysema, asthma, tuberclerosis

Comments: *Rings at caller's local chapter. Association offers BETTER BREATHING CLUBS, smoking cessation group clinics, school programs teaching lung health and smoking prevention, information, and referrals.

AMERICAN ORTHOTIC AND PROSTHETIC ASSOCIATION

1650 King St., #500
Alexandria, VA 22314
703–836–7116

Type of organization: professional
Public served: medical personnel

Offers: products
Disability/chronic illness: amputation

Comments: A professional association whose members work with amputees. Can give referrals on a local level.

AMERICAN PARALYSIS ASSOCIATION

500 Morris Ave.
Springfield, NJ 07081
1–800–225–0292
201–379–2690

Type of organization: nonprofit
Public served: researchers
Offers: research material
Disability/chronic illness: central nervous system injury or disease, resulting in paralysis

Comments: Raises money for research on spinal cord injuries. Also call APA Spinal Cord Injury Hotline at 1–800–526–3456 (U.S.) or 1–800–638–1733 (in MD).

AMERICAN PARKINSON'S DISEASE ASSOCIATION

60 Bay St., Ste. 401
Staten Island, NY 10301
1–800–223–2732
718–981–8001
FAX: 718–981–4399

17

Type of organization: nonprofit
Public served: individuals/families, general public, media, medical professionals, researchers
Offers: information, publication(s), support group(s), medical referrals, seminars/ workshops, research material
Disability/chronic illness: Parkinson's disease

Comments: Provides funds for research.

AMERICAN PRINTING HOUSE FOR THE BLIND
1839 Frankfort Ave.
P.O. Box 6085
Louisville, KY 40206–0085
1–800–223–1839
502–895–2405
FAX: 502–895–1509

Type of organization: nonprofit
Public served: individuals/families, general public, media, nonmedical professionals
Offers: information, reference material, publication(s), seminars/workshops
Disability/chronic illness: visual impairments

Comments: For the publication of literature in all media (braille, large type, recorded computer disk) for the blind and the manu-facture of educational aids for special use by visually impaired students, such as preschool and vocational materials and talking educational software. Sponsors educational research programs, Wings of Freedom Award, art contests, and has a museum of artifacts from the education field.

AMERICAN RADIO RELAY LEAGUE
225 Main St.
Newington, CT 06111–1494
203–666–1541
FAX: 203–665–7531

Type of organization: nonprofit
Public served: individuals/families, general public
Offers: information, publication(s), recreational opportunities
Disability/chronic illness: all

Comments: Gets non-ham operators involved with ham operators. Provides local contacts for those interested as well as information on various operating aids for those with disabilities.

AMERICAN RED CROSS, NATIONAL HEADQUARTERS
431 17th St. NW
Washington, DC 20006
202–737–8300

18

Type of organization: nonprofit
Public served: individuals/families, general public, media
Offers: information, publication(s), counseling
Disability/chronic illness: all

Comments: Has local chapters; services vary according to chapter size.

AMERICAN SOCIETY FOR DEAF CHILDREN

814 Thayer Ave.
Silver Spring, MD 20910
1-800-942-2732

Type of organization: nonprofit
Public served: individuals/families, general public, media, medical personnel
Offers: information, reference material, publication(s), support group(s), medical referrals, nonmedical referrals, seminars/workshops, civil rights assistance/advocacy
Disability/chronic illness: hearing impairments (in children)

Comments: Has local chapters; helps parents network with other parents.

AMERICAN SOCIETY OF HANDICAPPED PHYSICIANS

105 Morris Dr.
Bastrop, LA 71220
318-281-4436

Type of organization: professional
Public served: individuals/families, medical personnel
Offers: information, reference material, support group(s), consultations/guidance, civil rights assistance/advocacy
Disability/chronic illness: all

Comments: A forum and support group as well as legal and career counseling body for handicapped physicians. Provides information on resources, works against discrimination, and operates a speakers bureau and placement service.

AMERICAN SPEECH-LANGUAGE-HEARING ASSOCIATION

10801 Rockville Pike
Rockville, MD 20852
1-800-638-8255 (voice and TDD)*
301-897-5700 (voice or TDD)
FAX: 301-571-0457

Type of organization: nonprofit
Public served: individuals/families, general public, media, medical personnel, nonmedical professionals
Offers: information, publication(s), nonmedical referrals, seminars/workshops, research material
Disability/chronic illness: hearing impairments and speech disorders

Comments: *An information line.

AMERICAN STAIR-GLIDE CORPORATION
4001 East 138th St.
P.O. Box B
Grandview, MO 64030–2837
816–763–3100
FAX: 816–763–4467

Type of organization: private
Public served: individuals/families, general public
Offers: products
Disability/chronic illness: physical disabilities

Comments: Source for products for the handicapped; catalog available.

AMERICAN TRAUMA SOCIETY
8903 Presidential Pkwy.,
   Ste. 512
Upper Marlboro, MD
   20772–2656
1–800–556–7890
301–420–4189

Type of organization: nonprofit, professional
Public served: general public, medical personnel
Offers: education, publication(s), seminars/workshops
Disability/chronic illness: physical disabilities

Comments: Mission is to increase the public's awareness of trauma and prevention.

AMERICAN WHEELCHAIR BOWLING ASSOCIATION
Walt Roy
3620 Tamarack Dr.
Redding, CA 96003
916–241–6297
FAX: 916–244–6651

Type of organization: nonprofit
Public served: individuals/families
Offers: information, recreational opportunities

Disability/chronic illness: physical disabilities

Comments: Membership is $15 per year. Provides newsletter, specialty patches, contact with other wheelchair bowlers. Newsletter gives tournament information. National tournament held yearly.

AMIGA MOBILITY INTERNATIONAL
6693 Dixie Hwy.
Bridgeport, MI 48722
1–800–248–9131*
517–777–0910

Type of organization: private
Public served: individuals/families
Offers: products
Disability/chronic illness: physical disabilities

Comments: *Call for customer service; call 1–800–248–9130 for sales. Carries platform mobility aids and offers free brochures and information.

AMPUTEE SHOE AND GLOVE EXCHANGE
P.O. Box 27067
Houston, TX 77227

Type of organization: nonprofit
Public served: individuals/families
Offers: information, products

Disability/chronic illness: amputation

Comments: Free information exchange to facilitate swaps of shoes and gloves unneeded by amputees. Attempts to match amputees who need the opposite shoe or glove, who are about the same age and who have reasonably similar tastes. Open to men, women, and children.

AMPUTEES IN MOTION
P.O. Box 2703
Escondido, CA 92033
619–454–9300

Type of organization: nonprofit
Public served: individuals/families, medical personnel, nonmedical professionals
Offers: information, support group(s), counseling, recreational opportunities, rehabilitative services
Disability/chronic illness: amputation

Comments: Helps amputees of any age reestablish an active and satisfying life through visitation programs and civic, social, and recreational participation. Works with health care professionals in the regular rehabilitation program. Makes sporting and social activities available.

AMTRAK, NATIONAL RAILROAD PASSENGER CORPORATION

400 North Capitol St. NW
Washington, DC 20001
1–800–872–7245
202–383–3000

Type of organization: private
Public served: individuals/families, general public
Offers: travel assistance
Disability/chronic illness: mobility impairments

Comments: Can also call 1–800–523–6590 (TDD) or 1–800–562–6960 (in PA). Publishes *Access Amtrak;* can provide wheelchair assistance.

AMYOTROPHIC LATERAL SCLEROSIS

21021 Ventura Blvd., Ste. 321
Woodland Hills, CA 91364
1–800–782–4747
818–340–7500
FAX: 818–340–2060

Type of organization: nonprofit
Public served: individuals/families, general public, media, medical personnel, researchers
Offers: information, publication(s), support group(s), medical referrals, research material
Disability/chronic illness: amyotrophic lateral sclerosis (Lou Gehrig's disease)

Comments: Has local chapters.

ARC, ASSOCIATION FOR RETARDED CITIZENS OF THE UNITED STATES

500 East Border St., Ste. 300
Arlington, TX 76010
817–261–6003
817–277–0553 (TDD)
FAX: 817–277–3491

Type of organization: nonprofit
Public served: individuals/families, general public, media
Offers: information, reference material, publication(s), consultations/guidance, civil rights assistance/advocacy
Disability/chronic illness: mental retardation

Comments: Local chapters. Works on local, state, and national levels to promote services, research, public understanding, and legislation for mentally retarded persons and their families. Offers information and referral services, social programs, and training conferences.

ARTHRITIS FOUNDATION
1314 Spring St. NW
Atlanta, GA 30309–2898
404–872–7100
FAX: 404–872–0457

Type of organization: nonprofit
Public served: individuals/families, general public, media, medical personnel, researchers
Offers: information, reference material, publication(s), support group(s), counseling, medical referrals, seminars/workshops, research material
Disability/chronic illness: arthritis

Comments: Has local chapters.

ASSISTANCE DOGS INTERNATIONAL
c/o Robin Dickson
10175 Wheeler Rd.
Central Point, OR 97502
503–826–9220

Type of organization: nonprofit
Public served: individuals/families
Offers: information, education, products, living aids
Disability/chronic illness: visual impairments, hearing impairments, others

Comments: Centers for training hearing-ear dogs, seeing-eye dogs and other service dogs. Encourages cooperation among training centers and establishes standards of excellence.

ASSISTIVE DOGS OF AMERICA
8806 State Rte. 64
Swanton, OH 43558
419–825–3622

Type of organization: nonprofit
Public served: individuals/families, nonmedical professionals
Offers: information, education, products, living aids
Disability/chronic illness: mobility impairments, multiple physical disabilities, terminal illnesses

Comments: Provides specially trained dogs. Program is supported by individuals, corporations, civic and fraternal organizations, and dog and kennel clubs. Also runs a speakers bureau.

ASSISTIVE TECHNOLOGY CENTERS
119 First Ave.
Pittsburgh, PA 15222
1–800–247–5510
412–288–9441

Type of organization: private
Public served: individuals/families, medical personnel, intermediate parties
Offers: products

Disability/chronic illness: visual and hearing impairments

Comments: Works through rehabilitation centers; offers a catalog.

ASSOCIATED SERVICES FOR THE BLIND

919 Walnut St.
Philadelphia, PA 19107
215–627–0600
215–922–0692

Type of organization: nonprofit
Public served: individuals/families, general public, media
Offers: information, reference, publication(s), support group(s), counseling, nonmedical referrals, products, rehabilitative services, living aids, independent living assistance
Disability/chronic illness: visual impairments

Comments: A multiservice agency that provides services for blind and visually impaired people, allowing them to live independently. Activities include: a retail store carrying products for visually impaired, braille printing house, counseling service, radio reading service that reads newspapers and magazines over closed-circuit radio, referrals and job placement, speakers bureau, rehabilitation program.

ASSOCIATION FOR CHILDREN WITH DOWN SYNDROME

2616 Martin Ave.
Bellmore, NY 11710
516–221–4700
FAX: 516–221–4700

Type of organization: nonprofit, professional
Public served: individuals/families, medical personnel, nonmedical professionals
Offers: information, reference material, publication(s), support group(s), medical referrals, nonmedical referrals, seminars/workshops, recreational opportunities, civil rights assistance/advocacy, research material
Disability/chronic illness: Down syndrome

Comments: Has 1,000 members, who include parents of children with Down's syndrome and health and educational professionals. Acts as resource and information center. Works to maintain contact with the medical community and parents; attempts to dispel myths about the capabilities of afflicted children through Learning is Necessary to Care, an outreach program. Administers infant, toddler, and preschool programs in New York state. Offers recreational and socialization programs and support for children over 5 years of age and young adults.

ASSOCIATION FOR CHILDREN WITH RETARDED MENTAL DEVELOPMENT
162 Fifth Ave., 11th Fl.
New York, NY 10010
1-800-969-2276
212-741-0100
FAX: 212-627-8318

Type of organization: nonprofit
Public served: individuals/families, general public, media
Offers: information, diagnostic services, reference material, publication(s), support group(s), counseling, medical referrals, nonmedical referrals, seminars/workshops, recreational opportunities, civil rights assistance/advocacy, rehabilitative services, vocational services, independent living assistance
Disability/chronic illness: mental retardation and developmental disabilities

Comments: Centered in New York City area. Members include professionals, parents, siblings, and others interested in mentally re-

tarded and developmentally disabled children and adults. Offers programs for individuals, job placement, vocational rehabilitation centers, supported work programs, and advocacy for mentally retarded and developmentally disabled.

ASSOCIATION FOR HISPANIC HANDICAPPED OF NEW JERSEY
10 Jackson St.
Paterson, NJ 07501
201-279-0212

Type of organization: nonprofit
Public served: individuals/families
Offers: information, publication(s), support group(s), counseling, consultations/guidance, seminars/workshops, civil rights assistance/advocacy, vocational services
Disability/chronic illness: all

Comments: Serves Hispanic handicapped children and their parents; maintains a network of parents who share information on services. Their Parent Teaching Parent Program trains parents to be advocates for their children's rights. Offers vocational training and placement services. Although most members are in New Jersey, residents of all states are welcome and the development of similar programs is encouraged.

ASSOCIATION FOR REHABILITATION PROGRAMS IN DATA PROCESSING

P.O. Box 42787
Philadelphia, PA 19101–1787
301–640–5484

Type of organization: nonprofit
Public served: individuals/families, general public, media, non-medical professionals
Offers: information, reference material, publication(s), seminars/workshops, vocational services
Disability/chronic illness: all

Comments: Promotes rehabilitation programs in data processing, open to individuals, business and community leaders, and rehabilitation trainers.

ASSOCIATION FOR THE ADVANCEMENT OF BLIND AND RETARDED

164–09 Hillside Ave.
Jamaica, NY 11432
718–523–2222
FAX: 718–739–4750

Type of organization: nonprofit
Public served: individuals/families
Offers: information, nonmedical referrals, recreational services
Disability/chronic illness: multi-handicaps, visual impair-ments, mental retardation (in children)

Comments: Consists of community groups and individuals interested in helping multihandicapped blind and severely retarded adults. Has residences, treatment centers, and summer camps.

ASSOCIATION FOR THE EDUCATION AND REHABILITATION OF THE BLIND AND VISUALLY IMPAIRED

206 North Washington St., Ste. 320
Alexandria, VA 22314
703–548–1884

Type of organization: nonprofit, professional
Public served: individuals/families, general public, medical personnel, nonmedical professionals
Offers: information, publication(s), seminars/workshops, rehabilitative services, vocational services
Disability/chronic illness: visual impairments

Comments: Open to parents, educators, rehabilitators, administrators, agencies, schools, and others interested in education, guidance, vocational rehabilitation or occupational placement of visually impaired individuals. Works with colleges and universities on conferences and workshops. Has job placement services and a speakers bureau.

ASSOCIATION ON HIGHER EDUCATION AND DISABILITY
P.O. Box 21192
Columbus, OH 43221–0192
614–488–4972
FAX: 614–488–1172

Type of organization: nonprofit
Public served: individuals/families, nonmedical professionals
Offers: information, reference material, publication(s), non-medical referrals, consula-tions/guidance, civil rights assistance/advocacy, research material
Disability/chronic illness: all

Comments: Open to individuals in-terested in promoting the equal rights and opportunities of dis-abled postsecondary students, staff, faculty, and graduates. Pro-vides exchange of information for professionals in the field, con-ducts surveys on issues pertinent to disabled college students, and offers employment information on available positions.

ASTHMA & ALLERGY FOUNDATION OF AMERICA
1125 15th St. NW, #502
Washington, DC 20005
1–800–727–8462*
202–466–7643
FAX: 202–466–8940

Type of organization: nonprofit
Public served: individuals/families, general public, media, medical personnel, researchers
Offers: information, support group(s), medical referrals, research materials
Disability/chronic illness: asthma and allergies

Comments: *An information hot-line.

AUTISM SERVICES CENTER
Prichard Bldg., 605 9th St.
P.O. Box 507
Huntington, WV 25702
304–525–8014
FAX: 304–525–8026

Type of organization: nonprofit
Public served: individuals/families, general public, media
Offers: information, publica-tion(s), nonmedical referrals, civil rights assistance/ advocacy

Disability/chronic illness: autism, central nervous system disease or injury

Comments: Provides information to all callers as well as referrals to other resources. The Behavioral Center provides services only within a four-county area in Virginia.

AUTISM SOCIETY OF AMERICA

8601 Georgia Ave., Ste. 503
Silver Spring, MD 20910
1–800–3AUTISM
301–565–0433
FAX: 301–565–0834

Type of organization: nonprofit
Public served: individuals/families, general public, media, non-medical professionals
Offers: information, education, reference material, publication(s), support group(s), medical referrals, nonmedical referrals, seminars/workshops, civil rights assistance/advocacy, research material
Disability/chronic illness: autism

Comments: For parents, teachers, educators, psychologists, speech therapists, pediatric neurologists, and others interested in autism.

A/V HEALTH SERVICES, INC.

Cindy Collett-Hodges
P.O. Box 20271
Roanoke, VA 24018
703–389–4339

Type of organization: private
Public served: individuals/families, medical personnel, nonmedical professionals
Offers: recreational opportunities, products
Disability/chronic illness: physical disabilities

Comments: Sells video tapes on daily living activities, informational/motivational topics, and exercises.

AVKO EDUCATIONAL RESEARCH FOUNDATION

3084 West Willard Rd.
Birch Run, MI 48415
313–686–9283
FAX: 313–686–1101

Type of organization: nonprofit
Public served: individuals/families, general public
Offers: information, education, diagnostic services, reference material, publication(s), support group(s), counseling, seminars/workshops, research material

Disability/chronic illness: dyslexia and other learning disabilities

Comments: Members include teachers and others involved in helping others learn to read and spell and in developing reading training materials for those with dyslexia. Holds training sessions for family members who wish to teach reading and spelling to those with dyslexia. Offers community education classes, researches causes of dyslexia, maintains a library, and has a speakers bureau.

B

BARRIER FREE LIFTS
P.O. Box 4163
Manassas, VA 22110
1–800–582–8732
703–261–6531
FAX: 703–361–7861

Type of organization: private
Public served: individuals/families
Offers: products
Disability/chronic illness: physical disabilities

Comments: Brochures and videotapes of products available on request. Carries lifts to move physically disabled from bed to chair and in and out of the bath.

BEGINNINGS FOR PARENTS OF HEARING IMPAIRED CHILDREN
1504 Western Blvd.
Raleigh, NC 27606
1–800–541–4327
919–834–9100
FAX: 919–832–6990

Type of organization: government
Public served: individuals/families, general public, media
Offers: information, education, diagnostic services, reference material, publication(s), support group(s), counseling, medical referrals, nonmedical referrals, consultations/guidance, seminars/workshops, recreational opportunities, civil rights assistance/advocacy
Disability/chronic illness: hearing impairments (in children)

Comments: Previously a nonprofit organization; became part of North Carolina's Department of Human Resources in January 1994.

BETTER HEARING INSTITUTE
P.O. Box 1840
Washington, DC 20013
1–800–EAR–WELL*
703–642–0580
FAX: 703–750–9302

Type of organization: nonprofit
Public served: individuals/families, general public, media
Offers: information, publication(s), nonmedical referrals
Disability/chronic illness: hearing impairments

Comments: *In the U.S., except VA. Provides a list of resources.

BLIND CHILDREN CENTER
4120 Marathon St.
Los Angeles, CA 90029
1-800-222-3566
1-800-222-3567 (in CA)
FAX: 213-665-3828

Type of organization: nonprofit
Public served: individuals/families, general public, media, medical personnel, nonmedical professionals, researchers
Offers: information, education, diagnostic services, reference material, publication(s), support group(s), counseling, medical referrals, nommedical referrals, consultations/guidance, seminars/workshops, research material, rehabilitative services
Disability/chronic illness: visual impairments (in children, infants to 5 years of age)

Comments: Pen pal program and referrals open to any age.

BLIND SERVICE ASSOCIATION
22 West Monroe, 11th Fl.
Chicago, IL 60603
312-236-0808

Type of organization: nonprofit
Public served: individuals/families, general public
Offers: information, publication(s), financial assistance, recreational opportunities, products, living aids
Disability/chronic illness: visual impairments

Comments: Services include reading room for school, work-related and leisure material, field trips for blind students, cultural or recreational opportunities, recording of material on tapes, scholarship grants for blind college students, and some financial assistance in cooperation with other agencies in certain cases. Supports eye clinics, provides visual aids as needed.

BLINDED VETERANS ASSOCIATION
477 H St. NW
Washington, DC 20001
1-800-669-7079
202-371-8880
FAX: 202-371-8258

Type of organization: nonprofit
Public served: individuals/families
Offers: information, support group(s), counseling, rehabili-

tative services, vocational services

Disability/chronic illness: disabilities, visual impairments (in veterans)

Comments: Regular members are those whose blindness is considered service-connected; associates are veterans whose blindness is not service-connected. Aids regular members in obtaining veterans benefits, works to assist all in living well-adjusted, active, and productive lives.

BOOKS ON TAPE
729 Farad
Costa Mesa, CA 92627
1–800–626–3333

Type of organization: private
Public served: individuals/families
Offers: publication(s)
Disability/chronic illness: visual impairments

Comments: Brochure available for books that can be rented or purchased.

BOY SCOUTS OF AMERICA, SCOUTING FOR THE HANDICAPPED
135 Walnut Hill Ln.
Irving, TX 75038–3096
214–580–2000
FAX: 214–582–2502

Type of organization: nonprofit
Public served: individuals/families
Offers: information, recreational opportunities
Disability/chronic illness: all

Comments: Boys are in Cub Scout Packs or Boy Scout Troops while the Explorer Posts (high school age) are coed. Those with disabilities may be mainstreamed into regular troops and those with severe disabilities may be in special troops. Check for the local Boy Scout Council in the white pages of the telephone directory for more information. There are over 4,000 packs, troops, and posts for the disabled.

BRAILLE INSTITUTE OF AMERICA
741 North Vermont Ave.
Los Angeles, CA 90029
1–800–BRAILLE (in CA)
213–663–1111
FAX: 213–666–5881

Type of organization: nonprofit, private
Public served: individuals/families
Offers: information, education, counseling, rehabilitative services
Disability/chronic illness: visual impairments

Comments: Brochure available on request. This is an educational institute that serves students from infancy through high school.

BRAUN CORPORATION
1014 South Monticello
P.O. Box 310
Winamac, IN 46996
1–800–272–8611*
219–946–6157

Type of organization: private
Public served: individuals/families
Offers: products
Disability/chronic illness: physical
  disabilities

Comments: *This is the number for customer service (in the U.S., except MA). To order parts or reach the corporate office, call 1–800–272–8622 (in the U.S., except MA). Also sells wheelchair lifts.

BROWN LUNG ASSOCIATION
5461 Donna Rd.
Julian, NC 27283
919–685–9574

Type of organization: nonprofit
Public served: individuals/families
Offers: information, nonmedical
  referrals
Disability/chronic illness: brown
  lung (cotton dust injury to
  the lungs)

Comments: Referrals to lawyers are given.

BRS INFORMATION TECHNOLOGY
8000 Westpark Dr.
McLean, VA 22102
800–289–4277
703–556–6740 .
FAX: 703–893–4632

Type of organization: private
Public served: individuals/families,
  general public, media, medical
  personnel
Offers: information, reference
Disability/chronic illness: all

Comments: National database vendor providing medical information, some geared directly to medical professionals while others are directed toward individuals or the general public. Access is made available by subscription and usage fees. Call or write for more information.

C

CANCER CARE
1180 Avenue of the Americas
New York, NY 10036–8401
212–221–3300
FAX: 212–719–0263

Type of organization: nonprofit
Public served: individuals/families

Offers: information, education, reference material, publica-tion(s), support group(s), counseling, medical referrals, nonmedical referrals, consul-tations/guidance, seminars/workshops, financial assis-tance, civil rights assistance/advocacy, research material
Disability/chronic illness: cancer

Comments: A nonprofit social-service agency.

CANCER INFORMATION SERVICE, FLORIDA
Comprehensive Cancer Center
1475 Northwest 12th Ave.
P.O. Box 016960 (D8–4)
Miami, FL 33101
1–800–4–CANCER
305–548–6920

Type of organization: nonprofit, government
Public served: individuals/families, general public
Offers: information
Disability/chronic illness: cancer

Comments: In Oahu, HI, call 1–808–524–1234 (neighboring is-lands call collect). Call 1–800–638–6070 for answers to ques-tions about cancer in English and Spanish. Also offers publi-cations in English and some in Spanish.

CANCER NEWS MAGAZINE
1599 Clifton Rd. NE
Atlanta, GA 30329–4243
1–800–ACS–2345
404–320–3333
FAX: 404–325–2217

Type of organization: nonprofit
Public served: individuals/families, general public, media
Offers: information, publica-tion(s)
Disability/chronic illness: cancer

Comments: A magazine published by the American Cancer Soci-ety.

CANCER RESEARCH CENTER
3501 Berrywood Dr.
Columbia, MO 65201
314–875–2255
FAX: 314–443–1202

Type of organization: nonprofit, private research facility
Public served: medical personnel, researchers
Offers: research material (conducts research)
Disability/chronic illness: cancer

Comments: A research facility.

CANDLELIGHTERS CHILDHOOD CANCER FOUNDATION
7910 Woodmont Ave., #460
Bethesda, MD 20814
1–800–366–2223
301–657–8401
FAX: 301–718–2686

Type of organization: nonprofit
Public served: individuals/families, general public, media
Offers: information, reference material, publication(s), support group(s), counseling
Disability/chronic illness: pediatric cancer

Comments: An information clearinghouse and network of parents. Works to educate, support, serve, and be an advocate for families of children with cancer, survivors of childhood cancer, and the professionals who care for them.

CANINE COMPANIONS FOR INDEPENDENCE
P.O. Box 446
Santa Rosa, CA 95402–0446
707–528–0830
FAX: 707–528–0146

Type of organization: nonprofit
Public served: individuals/families, general public

Offers: information, publication(s), seminars/workshops, living aids
Disability/chronic illness: visual impairments, hearing impairments, and physical disabilities

Comments: Provides specially bred and trained dogs (Signal Dogs for hearing impaired, Social Dogs for pet therapy, and Service Dogs to provide personal assistance). Also provides training for individuals receiving the dogs.

CARROLL CENTER FOR THE BLIND
770 Centre St.
Newton, MA 02158
1–800–852–3131
617–969–6200
FAX: 617–969–6204

Type of organization: nonprofit
Public served: individuals/families, general public, media, nonmedical professionals
Offers: information, education, diagnostic services, reference material, publication(s), medical referrals, nonmedical referrals, seminars/workshops, products, rehabilitative services, independent living assistance

Disability/chronic illness: visual impairments

Comments: A rehabilitation center for adults 16 and up. Also trains workers through student internships and has a charitable program.

CENTER FOR FAMILY SUPPORT

386 Park Ave. South
New York, NY 10016
212–481–1082

Type of organization: nonprofit
Public served: individuals/families
Offers: information, support group(s), nonmedical referrals
Disability/chronic illness: mental retardation (in children)

Comments: A service agency devoted to the physical well-being and development of retarded children and the sound mental health of their parents. Helps families with retarded children with all aspects of home care, including counseling, referrals, home-aid service, and consultation. Offers intervention for parents after the birth of a retarded child with in-home support, guidance, and infant stimulation.

CENTERS FOR DISEASE CONTROL, DIABETES CONTROL PROGRAMS, OFFICE OF CHRONIC DISEASE PREVENTION AND HEALTH PROMOTION

CDC, 1600 Clifton Rd., EO8
Atlanta, GA 30333
404–639–1848

Type of organization: government
Public served: individuals/families
Offers: information, medical services
Disability/chronic illness: diabetes and its complications

CENTERS FOR DISEASE CONTROL, OFFICE OF PUBLIC AFFAIRS

1600 Clifton Rd.
Atlanta, GA 30333
404–639–3286

Type of organization: government
Public served: general public, media, medical personnel, researchers
Offers: information, publication(s), research material
Disability/chronic illness: all

Comments: Can provide literature on many health-related topics.

CEREBRAL PALSY RESEARCH FOUNDATION OF KANSAS

2021 North Old Manor
P.O. Box 8217
Wichita, KS 67208–0217
316–688–1888
FAX: 316–688–5687

Type of organization: nonprofit
Public served: individuals/families, medical personnel
Offers: information, education, diagnostic services, reference material, publication(s), support group(s), counseling, nonmedical referrals, consultations/guidance, seminars/workshops, financial assistance, recreational opportunities, civil rights assistance/advocacy, research material, living aids, rehabilitative services, vocational services, independent living assistance, housing
Disability/chronic illness: cerebral palsy, physical disabilities (infants to elderly)

Comments: A service provider that also researches workshop modification. Has a 100-unit HUD housing complex, and national rehabilitation engineering center with emphasis on workshop modification. Has manufacturing facilities in Wichita, KS, and Erlanger, KY (a Cincinnati, OH, suburb).

CHALLENGE INTERNATIONAL

1204 Ina Ln.
McLean, VA 22102
703–821–3385

Type of organization: nonprofit
Public served: individuals/families, general public, media
Offers: education, publication(s), consultations/guidance, civil rights assistance/advocacy
Disability/chronic illness: all

Comments: A media awareness campaign designed to make disability a familiar and comfortable issue by closing the gap between the general public and the disabled community. Purposes are to serve the disabled community by changing the way able Americans perceive disability and disabled individuals and to promote positive images of disabled persons in the media through newspaper articles, radio and television news reports, television shows, motion pictures, and advertisements; educate the public about disability-related issues; serve as a clearinghouse on the needs of the disabled and the organizations that represent them; assist the media so they realistically and appropriately report on disability and disabled persons; and encourage the acceptance of people with disabilities, enabling them to become more productive members of society.

CHILDREN'S EMOTIONS ANONYMOUS

c/o Martha Bush
P.O. Box 4245
St. Paul, MN 55104-0245
612-647-9712
FAX: 612-647-1593

Type of organization: nonprofit
Public served: individuals/families
Offers: support group(s), counseling
Disability/chronic illness: mental illness (in children)

Comments: A program of Emotions Anonymous for children ages 5 to 12 that helps members develop strong emotional health, a positive attitude, and the ability to cope with personal problems. Uses the Twelve Steps of Alcoholics Anonymous World Services, which are adapted to pertain to children's emotional problems. Conducts weekly discussion group led by an adult member of EA.

CHILDREN'S HOSPITAL

Library
P.O. Box 14871
400 South Kings Hwy. Blvd.
St. Louis, MO 63178
314-454-6000

Type of organization: medical facility
Public served: individuals/families, general public, media, medical personnel
Offers: information, reference material
Disability/chronic illness: all (in children)

Comments: Pediatric and nursing literature available.

CHILDREN'S MEMORIAL HOSPITAL

Division of Genetics
2300 Children's Plaza
Chicago, IL 60614
312-880-4462

Type of organization: medical facility
Public served: individuals/families, medical personnel
Offers: information, diagnostic services, reference material, medical services
Disability/chronic illness: genetic disorders

Comments: At press time, only patients with genetic metabolism problems were being seen because only one geneticist was available. However, the hospital was searching for another doctor.

CHRISTIAN RECORD SERVICES
4444 South 52nd St.
Lincoln, NE 68516
402–488–7582

Type of organization: nonprofit
Public served: individuals/families
Offers: information, reference material, publication(s), counseling, financial assistance, products
Disability/chronic illness: visual and hearing impairments

Comments: Has a lending library of videotapes, braille books, books on cassette and books in large print. Has *Bible* correspondence courses, visitation activities, some limited scholarship or financial assistance; holds glaucoma screening clinics and some camps for youth.

CHRONIC FATIGUE IMMUNE DYSFUNCTION SYNDROME (CFIDS) ASSOCIATION
P.O. Box 220398
Charlotte, NC 28222
1–800–442–3437

Type of organization: nonprofit
Public served: individuals/families, general public, media, medical personnel
Offers: information, reference material, publication(s), support group(s), counseling, medical referrals
Disability/chronic illness: chronic fatigue (CFIDS)

Comments: Also operates an information line (900–896–2343), which costs $2 for the first minute and $1 for each additional minute.

CLEARINGHOUSE OF OCCUPATIONAL SAFETY & HEALTH INFORMATION, NATIONAL INSTITUTE OF OCCUPATIONAL SAFETY & HEALTH
200 Independence Ave. SW
Washington, DC 20201
1–800–356–4674
202–690–7134
FAX: 202–690–7519

Type of organization: government
Public served: individuals/families, general public, media
Offers: information
Disability/chronic illness: cancer

Comments: Produces publications that indicate products with carcinogens.

COMMITTEE FOR PURCHASE FROM THE BLIND AND OTHER SEVERELY HANDICAPPED

1735 Jefferson Davis Hwy., #403
Arlington, VA 22202
703–603–7740
FAX: 703–412–7113

Type of organization: government
Public served: individuals/families
Offers: vocational assistance
Disability/chronic illness: visual impairments, severe handicaps

Comments: Acts as a liaison between federal government purchasing offices and workshops.

CONGRESS OF ORGANIZATIONS OF THE PHYSICALLY HANDICAPPED

16630 Beverly Ave.
Tinley Park, IL 60477–1904
708–532–3566

Type of organization: nonprofit
Public served: individuals/families, nonmedical professionals, intermediate parties
Offers: information, consultations/guidance, civil rights assistance/advocacy
Disability/chronic illness: physical disabilities

Comments: Members are organizations that provide services to physically disabled: serves as liaison between members and professional organizations.

COOLEY'S ANEMIA FOUNDATION

105 East 22nd St., Ste. 911
New York, NY 10010
1–800–221–3571
1–800–522–7222 (in NY)
FAX: 212–598–4892

Type of organization: nonprofit
Public served: individuals/families, general public, media, medical personnel
Offers: information, reference material, publication(s), support group(s), counseling, medical referrals, research material
Disability/chronic illness: Cooley's anemia

Comments: Can also be reached at 212–598–0911.

CORNELIA DE LANGE SYNDROME FOUNDATION

60 Dyer Ave.
Collinsville, CT 06022
1–800–223–8355
203–693–0159
FAX: 203–693–6819

Type of organization: nonprofit
Public served: individuals/families, general public, media, medical

personnel, nonmedical professionals

Offers: information, publica-
tion(s), support group(s),
medical referrals, research
material

Disability/chronic illness: Cornelia
de Lange syndrome

Comments: Regional coordinators
who reach out to people. A network of families who have a child
with the syndrome.

COUNCIL OF CITIZENS WITH LOW VISION

1400 North Drake Rd.,
No. 218
Kalamazoo, MI 49007
1-800-733-2258
616-381-9566

Type of organization: nonprofit

Public served: individuals/families,
nonmedical professionals

Offers: information, education,
publication(s), support
group(s), nonmedical referrals,
civil rights assistance/advo-
cacy, research material,
products, independent
living assistance

Disability/chronic illness: visual
impairments

Comments: Partially sighted and
low-vision individuals, their families, and professional workers.

Promotes the development of fullest potential of those with some
sight. Gives them a forum to discuss their needs, preferences, and
interests. Seeks utilization of any
visual aid, service, or technology
for maximizing the sight they do
have. Keeps members abreast of
latest developments that will benefit them.

COUNCIL FOR EXCEPTIONAL CHILDREN (SPECIAL EDUCATION)

1920 Association Dr.
Reston, VA 22091-1589
703-620-3660
FAX: 703-264-9494

Type of organization: nonprofit,
professional

Public served: individuals/families,
general public, media, nonmedical professionals,
intermediate parties

Offers: information, education,
publication(s), medical referrals, nonmedical referrals, con-
sultations/guidance, seminars/
workshops, civil rights assis-
tance/advocacy

Disability/chronic illness: developmental disabilities, mental
retardation, visual and hearing
impairments, physical and
learning disabilities, speech
defects, behavioral disorders

Comments: Promotes education for any children whose needs fall outside the "average" level of education. This applies to mentally gifted as well as handicapped. Open to parents, teachers, administrators, and others. Has several divisions, including ERIC database.

CYSTIC FIBROSIS FOUNDATION
6931 Arlington Rd.
Bethesda, MD 20814
1–800–344–4823
301–951–4422
FAX: 301–951–6378

Type of organization: nonprofit
Public served: individuals/families, general public, media, medical personnel, researchers
Offers: information, support group(s), counseling, medical referrals
Disability/chronic illness: cystic fibrosis

Comments: Has local chapters.

D

DEAFNESS RESEARCH FOUNDATION
9 East 38th St., 7th Fl.
New York, NY 10016
1–800–535–3323
212–684–6556
FAX: 212–779–2125

Type of organization: nonprofit
Public served: individuals/families, general public, medical personnel
Offers: information, publication(s), medical referrals, research material
Disability/chronic illness: hearing impairments

Comments: Through its financial support of medical research and the dissemination of information to the public sector, improves the quality of life for the nation's 28 million who are deaf, profoundly hearing impaired, or are affected by other serious ear disorders.

DEPRESSIVES ANONYMOUS: RECOVER FROM DEPRESSION
329 East 62nd St.
New York, NY 10021
213–268–7220

Type of organization: nonprofit
Public served: individuals/families
Offers: support group(s), counseling
Disability/chronic illness: mental illness, depression

Comments: Fellowship of men and women who gather together to help each other recover from emotional problems or illness, and to grow emotionally and spiritually. Seeks to help emotionally troubled individuals during and after their times of crisis. Operates through self-help groups and follows a modified version of the Twelve Steps of Alcoholics Anonymous World Services.

DIABETES RESEARCH INSTITUTE FOUNDATION

8600 Northwest 53rd Terrace, Ste. 202
Miami, FL 33166
1-800-321-3437
305-477-3437
FAX: 305-593-0439

Type of organization: nonprofit
Public served: individuals/families, general public, media
Offers: information, publication(s), research material
Disability/chronic illness: diabetes

DIABETES TREATMENT CENTER OF AMERICA

One Virgin Hills Blvd., Ste. 300
Nashville, TN 37215
1-800-327-3822
615-665-1133
FAX: 615-665-7697

Type of organization: private, medical facility
Public served: individuals/families
Offers: information, medical referrals, medical services
Disability/chronic illness: diabetes

Comments: Has treatment centers across the U.S.

DISABILITY RIGHTS CENTER

2500 Q St. NW, #121
Washington, DC 20007
202-337-4119

Type of organization: nonprofit
Public served: individuals/families, general public, media, nonmedical professionals
Offers: information, reference material, publication(s), civil rights assistance/advocacy
Disability/chronic illness: all

Comments: Public-interest research group committed to protecting and enforcing the legal rights of disabled citizens. Not open to membership but does offer publications.

DISABILITY RIGHTS EDUCATION AND DEFENSE FUND

2212 Sixth St.
Berkeley, CA 94710
510-644-2555*
FAX: 510-841-8645

Type of organization: nonprofit
Public served: individuals/families, general public, media
Offers: information, publication(s), consultations/guidance, civil rights assistance/

advocacy, rehabilitative services, vocational services
Disability/chronic illness: all

Comments: *Also 510–644–2626 (TDD). Focuses on advocacy for civil rights of those with disabilities.

DISABLED AMERICAN VETERANS
807 Maine Ave. SW
Washington, DC 20024
202–554–3501

Type of organization: nonprofit
Public served: individuals/families
Offers: information, reference material, publication(s), support group(s), counseling, non-medical referrals, civil rights assistance/advocacy
Disability/chronic illness: disabilities (in veterans)

Comments: Works with disabled veterans in obtaining benefits from the Veterans Administration. Local offices at most VA facilities or local chapters.

DU-IT CONTROL SYSTEMS GROUP
8765 Township Rd., No. 513
Shreve, OH 44676
216–567–2001
FAX: 216–567–3925

Type of organization: private
Public served: individuals/families
Offers: information, products, living aids
Disability/chronic illness: physical disabilities

Comments: Company produces high-tech controls for wheelchairs, lifts, and such environmental items as lights, drapes, heating, and cooling. They design and manufacture these items for the extremely physically disabled, such as victims of multiple sclerosis, muscular dystrophy, ALS (Lou Gehrig's disease), high-level spinal cord injuries, or stroke. They generally work through rehabilitation professionals.

E

EASTERN PARALYZED VETERANS ASSOCIATION
75–20 Astoria Bldg.
Jackson Heights, NY 11370–1177
718–803–3782
FAX: 718–803–0414

Type of organization: nonprofit
Public served: individuals/families
Offers: information, reference material, publication(s), non-medical referrals, seminars/

43

workshops, civil rights assis-
tance/advocacy
Disability/chronic illness: disabilities, central nervous system
disease and injury

Comments: Serves as a resource
center for veterans and nonveterans with spinal cord injuries, or
anyone who has problems with accessibility. They can answer ques-
tions regarding state laws and the
Americans with Disabilities Act.

ELECTRONIC UNIVERSITY NETWORK
1977 Colestin Rd.
Hornbrook, CA 96044
1–800–225–3276
503–482–5871
FAX: 503–482–7544

Type of organization: private
Public served: individuals/families
Offers: education
Disability/chronic illness: all

Comments: Facilitator that offers
classes handled with a computer
and modem.

EMOTIONS ANONYMOUS
P.O. Box 4245
St. Paul, MN 55104–0245
612–647–9712
FAX: 612–647–1593

Type of organization: nonprofit
Public served: individuals/families

Offers: publication(s), support
group(s), counseling
Disability/chronic illness: mental
illness

Comments: Over 1,300 local
groups. A "fellowship of men and
women who share their experience, strength and hope with each
other, that they may solve their
common problem and help others
recover from emotional illness."
Uses the Twelve Steps of Alcoholics Anonymous World Services
adapted to emotional problems.
Disseminates literature and information, provides telephone referrals to local groups.

EPILEPSY FOUNDATION OF AMERICA
4351 Garden City Dr.
Landover, MD 20785
1–800–EFA–1000*
301–459–3700
FAX: 301–577–2684

Type of organization: nonprofit
Public served: individuals/families,
general public, media, medical
personnel, researchers
Offers: information, reference material, publication(s), support
group(s), counseling, medical
referrals, medical services,
civil rights assistance/advo-
cacy, research material
Disability/chronic illness: epilepsy

Comments: *In U.S., except AK and HI where residents should call 1–800–332–6662. Has local chapters.

EVEREST & JENNINGS
3233 Mission Oaks Blvd.
Camarillo, CA 93010
805–987–6911

Type of organization: private
Public served: individuals/families
Offers: products
Disability/chronic illness: physical disabilities

Comments: A producer of wheelchairs.

EXTENSIONS FOR INDEPENDENCE
555 Saturn Blvd., B-368
San Diego, CA 92154
619–423–7709

Type of organization: private
Public served: individuals/families, general public, media
Offers: information, reference material, consultations/guidance, products, living aids
Disability/chronic illness: physical disabilities

Comments: Develops, manufactures, and markets vocational equipment for the physically disabled. Promotes improvements in design, materials, production, and quality of products while maintaining affordable prices.

F

FAMILY RESOURCE CENTER ON DISABILITIES
20 East Jackson, Rm. 900
Chicago, IL 60604
312–939–3513
FAX: 312–939–7297

Type of organization: nonprofit, private
Public served: individuals/families, general public, media
Offers: information, reference material, publication(s), counseling, medical referrals, nonmedical referrals, seminars/workshops
Disability/chronic illness: all

Comments: Teaches parents how to obtain needed services for their disabled children by knowing the laws pertaining to special education and services. Workshops held every Tuesday morning.

FAMILY SERVICE ASSOCIATION OF AMERICA
11700 West Lake Park Dr.
Milwaukee, WI 53224
1–800–221–2681
414–359–1040
FAX: 414–359–1074

Type of organization: nonprofit, professional
Public served: individuals/families
Offers: counseling
Disability/chronic illness: any, or none

Comments: Contact them for referral to a nearby agency for counseling.

FEDERATION FOR CHILDREN WITH SPECIAL NEEDS
95 Berkley St., Ste. 104
Boston, MA 02116
1–800–331–0688 (in MA)
617–482–2915
FAX: 617–695–2939

Type of organization: nonprofit
Public served: individuals/families, general public, media, medical personnel, nonmedical professionals
Offers: information, reference material, publication(s), counseling, consultations/guidance, seminars/workshops
Disability/chronic illness: developmental disabilities (in children and adults)

Comments: A coalition of parents. Organization provides information on special education laws and resources and on how to obtain related services. Promotes parents' active involvement in health care and provides assistance to parents. Although membership is primarily in New England, activities are national in scope.

FIBROMYALGIA ASSOCIATION OF CENTRAL OHIO
Riverside Hospital
3545 Olentangy River Rd., Ste. 8
Columbus, OH 43214
614–262–2000

Type of organization: nonprofit
Public served: individuals/families, general public, media, medical personnel, nonmedical professionals
Offers: information, reference material, publication(s), support groups, medical referrals, nonmedical referrals, seminars/workshops
Disability/chronic illness: fibromyalgia

FIBROMYALGIA ASSOCIATION OF FLORIDA, INC.
P.O. Box 14848
Gainesville, FL 32604–4848
904–371–2750

Type of organization: nonprofit
Public served: individuals/families, general public, media, medical personnel
Offers: information, publication(s), support group(s), medical referrals, seminars/workshops

46

Disability/chronic illness: fibromyalgia

Comments: Made up of local chapters throughout Florida.

FIBROMYALGIA ASSOCIATION OF TEXAS, INC.
5650 Forest Ln.
Dallas, TX 75230
214–363–2473

Type of organization: nonprofit
Public served: individuals/families, general public, media, medical personnel
Offers: information, publication(s), support group(s), medical referrals, nonmedical referrals
Disability/chronic illness: fibro-
myalgia

FOUNDATION FOR SCIENCE AND THE HANDICAPPED
236 Grand St.
Morgantown, WV 26505–7509
304–293–5201

Type of organization: professional organization
Public served: individuals/families, general public, medical personnel, nonmedical professionals
Offers: information, reference material, consultations/guidance, financial assistance, vocational services

Disability/chronic illness: physical disabilities

Comments: Disabled scientists and interested individuals. Offers consultation and advice concerning problems faced by handicapped persons in scientific fields. Provides grants to disabled graduate or professional school students in engineering, science, and health-related areas.

FOUNDATION FOR THE STUDY OF WILSON'S DISEASE
5447 Palisade Ave.
Bronx, NY 10471
718–430–2091

Type of organization: research facility
Public served: individuals/families, general public, media, medical personnel
Offers: information, reference material, research material
Disability/chronic illness: Wilson's disease, liver disease

Comments: A research facility.

FREEDOM DRIVING AIDS, INC.
Handicapped Drivers
Mobility Center
23855 West Andrew Rd.
Plainfield, IL 60544
1–800–843–0511*
815–254–2000

47

Type of organization: private
Public served: individuals/families
Offers: travel assistance, products
Disability/chronic illness: physical disabilities

Comments: *In IL and MI (517 area code only), or 1–800–321–7736 in MI and IL (815 area code only).

FREEDOM WHEELCHAIR LIFTS, INC.
1080 Katy Rd.
Keller, TX 76248
817–431–9437

Type of organization: private
Public served: individuals/families
Offers: products
Disability/chronic illness: physical disabilities

Comments: They modify vans by installing lifts for those in wheelchairs.

G

GALLAUDET COLLEGE
7th and Florida Ave. NE
Washington, DC 20002
1–800–451–8834
202–651–5100

Type of organization: college/university
Public served: individuals/families, general public, media, medical personnel, researchers

Offers: information, counseling, medical referrals, civil rights assistance/advocacy, research material, rehabilitative services, vocational services
Disability/chronic illness: hearing impairments

Comments: University that serves hearing-impaired individuals. Provides information on many aspects of deafness and communication methods. See additional listings.

GALLAUDET COLLEGE, ADULT BASIC EDUCATION PROGRAM
800 Florida Ave. NE
Washington, DC 20002
1–800–451–8834*
202–651–5000

Type of organization: college/university
Public served: individuals/families
Offers: information
Disability/chronic illness: hearing impairments

Comments: *The college's main number.

GALLAUDET COLLEGE, NATIONAL CENTER FOR LAW AND THE DEAF
7th St. and Florida Ave. NE
Washington, DC 20002
1–800–451–8834*

Type of organization: college/
university
Public served: individuals/families
Offers: information, civil rights
assistance/advocacy
Disability/chronic illness: hearing
impairments

Comments: *The college's main
number. Provides legal advice,
publications list.

GALLAUDET COLLEGE, THE NATIONAL INFORMATION CENTER ON DEAFNESS
800 Florida Ave. NE
Washington, DC 20002
1–800–451–8834*
202–651–5109

Type of organization: college/
university
Public served: individuals/families,
general public, media
Offers: information
Disability/chronic illness: hearing
impairments

Comments: *The college's main
number.

GALLAUDET RESEARCH INSTITUTE, SIGNED ENGLISH PROJECT, CENTER FOR STUDIES IN EDUCATION AND HUMAN DEVELOPMENT
Washington, DC 20002
1–800–451–8834*
202–651–5281

Type of organization: college/
university
Public served: individuals/families,
general public
Offers: information, education,
publication(s)
Disability/chronic illness: hearing
impairments

Comments: *The college's main
number. Does consulting.

GAZETTE INTERNATIONAL NETWORKING INSTITUTION (GINI)
5100 Oakland Ave., No. 206
St. Louis, MO 63110
314–534–0475

Type of organization: nonprofit
Public served: individuals/families,
general public, media, medical
personnel, nonmedical
professionals
Offers: information, education,
reference material, publica-
tion(s), support group(s),
counseling, seminars/
workshops
Disability/chronic illness: polio and
spinal cord injuries, neuromuscular diseases, others
causing need for ventilator

Comments: Communication network to provide information to
those with polio, spinal cord injuries, neuromuscular diseases as
well as their health care person-

nel, insurance agencies, government agencies, independent living centers, and anyone else interested. Serves as a clearinghouse for information. Several publications, including a post-polio directory, are available.

GIRL SCOUTS OF THE USA, SCOUTING FOR THE HANDICAPPED
830 Third Ave.
New York, NY 10022
212–940–7500

Type of organization: nonprofit
Public served: individuals/families
Offers: information, recreational opportunities
Disability/chronic illness: all

Comments: Those with disabilities may be mainstreamed into regular troops and those with severe disabilities may be in special troops. Check with the local Girl Scout Council for more information.

GOODWILL INDUSTRIES OF AMERICA
9200 Wisconsin Ave.
Bethesda, MD 20814
301–530–6500*
FAX: 301–530–1516

Type of organization: nonprofit
Public served: individuals/families

Offers: information, publication(s), rehabilitative services, vocational services
Disability/chronic illness: physical disabilities, mental retardation

Comments: *Also 301–530–9759 (TDD). Concerned primarily with providing employment, training, evaluation, counseling, placement, and other vocational rehabilitation services and opportunities for personal growth to disabled and vocationally disadvantaged people.

GREYHOUND LINES, THE HELPING HAND SERVICES FOR THE HANDICAPPED
Section S, Greyhound Tower
Phoenix, AZ 85077
1–800–345–3109*

Type of organization: private
Public served: general public
Offers: travel assistance
Disability/chronic illness: all

Comments: *In the U.S., except NC. In NC call 1–800–342–6214.

GUIDE DOG FOUNDATION FOR THE BLIND
371 East Jericho Tnpk.
Smithtown, NY 11787
1–800–548–4337
516–265–2121
FAX: 516–361–5192

Type of organization: nonprofit
Public served: individuals/families
Offers: products, living aids
Disability/chronic illness: visual impairments

Comments: Provides trained dogs for those who qualify as visually impaired, along with training assistance for individuals (26 days) and free assistance for life. Also has speakers bureau.

GUIDE DOGS FOR THE BLIND

350 Los Ranchitos Rd.
P.O. Box 1200
San Rafael, CA 94915
415–479–4000

Type of organization: nonprofit
Public served: individuals/families, general public
Offers: information, reference material, publication(s), non-medical referrals, living aids
Disability/chronic illness: visual impairments

GUIDE DOGS OF AMERICA

13445 Glenoaks Blvd.
Sylmar, CA 91342
818–362–5834
FAX: 818–362–6870

Type of organization: nonprofit
Public served: individuals/families

Offers: education, products, living aids
Disability/chronic illness: visual impairments

Comments: Trains guide dogs and their new owners at no charge.

GUIDING EYES FOR THE BLIND

611 Granite Springs Rd.
Yorktown Heights, NY 10598
914–245–4024
FAX: 914–245–1609

Type of organization: nonprofit
Public served: individuals/families, general public, nonmedical professionals
Offers: information, education, seminars/workshops, products, living aids
Disability/chronic illness: visual impairments

Comments: Provides guide dogs and training for the blind. Conducts training for instructors. Has speakers bureau.

H

HANDICAP INTRODUCTIONS

1215 Brigantine Rd.
Manahawkin, NJ 08050
609–660–0606

Type of organization: nonprofit
Public served: individuals/families
Offers: information, recreational opportunities
Disability/chronic illness: all

Comments: A group of handicapped and nonhandicapped individuals for whom physical disability poses no barrier to an active social life. Seeks to introduce persons who are likely to be compatible in a dating relationship. Offers individual counseling; maintains speakers bureau and database of member profiles.

HANDICAPPED SCUBA ASSOCIATION

7172 West Stanford Ave.
Littleton, CO 80123
303–933–4864

Type of organization: nonprofit
Public served: individuals/families
Offers: education, recreational opportunities
Disability/chronic illness: physical disabilities

Comments: Promotes scuba diving by the handicapped. Membership open to both handicapped and able-bodied. Provides instructors and training, and coordinates four diving vacations a year. Has database of instructors.

HEADACHE RESEARCH FOUNDATION

c/o The Faulkner Hospital
Allandale at Centre St.
Jamaica Plain, MA 02130
617–522–7900*

Type of organization: medical facility, research facility
Public served: individuals/families, general public, media, medical personnel
Offers: information, reference material, medical referrals, consultations/guidance, research material
Disability/chronic illness: headaches

Comments: *For the educational division, or 617–522–6969 for research and patient care divisions.

HEARTLIFE

P.O. Box 54305
Atlanta, GA 30308
1–800–241–6993
404–523–0826

Type of organization: nonprofit
Public served: individuals/families
Offers: information, support group(s)
Disability/chronic illness: cardiac conditions

Comments: Helps local chapters organize.

HELEN KELLER NATIONAL CENTER FOR DEAF-BLIND YOUTHS AND ADULTS

111 Middle Neck Rd.
Sands Point, NY 11050
516–944–8900

Type of organization: medical facility, research facility
Public served: individuals/families, general public, medical personnel
Offers: information, reference material, medical referrals, rehabilitative services
Disability/chronic illness: hearing, visual impairments

HIGHER EDUCATION AND THE HANDICAPPED (HEATH)

One Dupont Cr. NW, Ste. 800
Washington, DC 20036
1–800–544–3284
202–939–9320
FAX: 202–833–4760

Type of organization: nonprofit
Public served: individuals/families, general public, media, non-medical professionals, intermediate parties
Offers: information, education, publication(s), counseling, financial assistance, vocational services, independent living assistance
Disability/chronic illness: all

Comments: A program of the American Council on Education that seeks to inform and assist disabled students continuing with postsecondary education. Works with educational institutions' administrators, educators, and disabled students. Also runs the National Clearinghouse on Post-Secondary Education for Handicapped Individuals. List of publications available. Promotes scholarships.

HORIZONS FOR THE BLIND

7001 North Clark St.
Chicago, IL 60626
312–973–7600

Type of organization: nonprofit
Public served: individuals/families
Offers: information, consultations/guidance, recreational opportunities
Disability/chronic illness: visual impairments

HUXLEY INSTITUTE/ AMERICAN SCHIZOPHRENIA ASSOCIATION

900 North Federal Hwy.
Boca Raton, FL 33432
1–800–847–3802
305–393–6167

Type of organization: nonprofit
Public served: individuals/families, general public, media, medical personnel
Offers: information, medical referrals
Disability/chronic illness: schizophrenia, manic depression, other mental illnesses

Comments: Reference collection is available for on-site study.

I

INDOOR SPORTS CLUB
1145 Highland St.
Napoleon, OH 43545
419–592–5756

Type of organization: nonprofit
Public served: individuals/families
Offers: information, education, support group(s), recreational opportunities, rehabilitative services
Disability/chronic illness: physical disabilities

Comments: A social, benevolent, educational, and rehabilitative organization that seeks to provide entertainment and amusement for disabled persons and shut-ins. Seeks aid for those in need and provides opportunities for involve-ment in civic affairs. Has 11 regional and 84 local groups.

INNOVATIVE REHABILITATION TECHNOLOGY, INC.
1411 West El Camino Real
Mountain View, CA 94040
1–800–322–4784
415–961–3161

Type of organization: private
Public served: individuals/families, general public, media
Offers: products
Disability/chronic illness: visual impairments

Comments: Publishes the *Technical Innovations Bulletin*.

INSTITUTE FOR BASIC RESEARCH IN DEVELOPMENTAL DISABILITIES
1050 Forest Hill Rd.
Staten Island, NY 10314
718–494–0600

Type of organization: research facility
Public served: medical personnel
Offers: reference material, research material
Disability/chronic illness: Alzheimer's disease, Down's syndrome, other neuro-degenerative diseases

INSTITUTE FOR REHABILITATION AND RESEARCH INFORMATION SERVICE CENTER

P.O. Box 20095
Houston, TX 77225
713-797-5947

Type of organization: research
  facility
Public served: individuals/families,
  general public, media, medical
  personnel, nonmedical
  professionals, researchers
Offers: information, reference
  material, research material
Disability/chronic illness: spinal
  cord injuries, amputations,
  neurological disorders,
  respiratory diseases both in
  children and adults

Comments: Facility is primarily
for adults, but also has a pediatric
ward.

INSTITUTE FOR RESEARCH OF RHEUMATIC DISEASES

Ansonia Station, Box 955
New York, NY 10023
212-595-1368

Type of organization: research
  facility
Public served: individuals/families,
  general public, media, medical
  personnel

Offers: information, reference
  material, publication(s)
Disability/chronic illness: arthritis

Comments: Promotes holistic approach to treatment for arthritis.

INSTITUTE OF LOGOPEDICS

2400 Jardine Dr.
Wichita, KS 67219
1-800-835-1043

Type of organization: nonprofit
Public served: individuals/families,
  general public
Offers: information, medical
  services, research material
Disability/chronic illness: multiple
  handicaps (in children)

Comments: Provides diagnostic,
therapeutic, educational, and social development services, plus information.

INSTITUTE OF REHABILITATION MEDICINE

400 East 34th St.
New York, NY 10016
212-340-6200

Type of organization: research
  facility
Public served: individuals/families,
  medical personnel
Offers: information, reference
  material, publication(s), medical services, consultations/

guidance, seminars/work-
shops, rehabilitative
services
Disability/chronic illness: all physical disabilities

INTERNATIONAL ASSOCIATION OF LARYNGECTOMEES

c/o American Cancer Society
1599 Clifton Rd. NE
Atlanta, GA 30329
404–320–3333

Type of organization: nonprofit
Public served: individuals/families,
general public, media, medical
personnel, nonmedical
professionals
Offers: information, publica-
tion(s), support group(s),
seminars/workshops
Disability/chronic illness: loss
of vocal chords through
laryngectomy

Comments: Open to individuals as
well as health professionals and
others interested in the rehabilitation of laryngectomees.

INTERNATIONAL CYSTIC FIBROSIS ASSOCIATION

3567 East 49th St.
Cleveland, OH 44105
216–271–1100

Type of organization: nonprofit
Public served: individuals/families,
general public, media, medical
personnel
Offers: information, reference
material, support group(s),
research material
Disability/chronic illness: cystic
fibrosis

INTERNATIONAL INSTITUTE FOR VISUALLY IMPAIRED

1975 Rutgers Cr.
East Lansing, MI 48823
517–332–2666

Type of organization: nonprofit
Public served: individuals/families,
nonmedical professionals
Offers: information, education,
reference material, publica-
tion(s), seminars/workshops
Disability/chronic illness: visual
impairments (in preschool
children only)

Comments: Clearinghouse for information and training.

INTERNATIONAL RETT'S SYNDROME ASSOCIATION

8511 Rose Marie Dr.
Fort Washington, MD 20744
301–248–7031

Type of organization: nonprofit
Public served: individuals/families,
researchers

Offers: information, reference material, publication(s), support group(s)
Disability/chronic illness: Rett's syndrome, genetic disorders

INTERNATIONAL WHEELCHAIR AVIATORS
Bill Blackwood
1117 Rising Hill Way
Escondido, CA 92029
619–746–5018

Type of organization: nonprofit
Public served: individuals/families, general public
Offers: recreational opportunities
Disability/chronic illness: physical disabilities

Comments: Offers information on how to get training, certification to fly. Has fly-ins in California. Has 200-plus members worldwide. Has newsletter. $15 a year for membership. Information is free.

INTERNATIONAL WHEELCHAIR ROAD RACERS CLUB, INC.
c/o Joseph M. Dowling
30 Myano Ln., Box 3
Stamford, CT 06902
203–967–2231

Type of organization: nonprofit
Public served: individuals/families, general public
Offers: information, recreational opportunities
Disability/chronic illness: physical disability

Comments: Involves physically disabled racers, able-bodied persons, rehabilitation institutes, and major road-race organizations in promoting wheelchair road racing in the U.S. Provides educational and technical support, maintains network of wheelchair road racers.

J

JAMES WHITCOMB RILEY HOSPITAL FOR CHILDREN, RILEY CHILD DEVELOPMENT PROGRAM
702 Barnhill Dr.
Indianapolis, IN 46223
317–264–4464

Type of organization: medical facility, research facility
Public served: individuals/families, medical personnel
Offers: information, education, medical referrals, medical services, research material
Disability/chronic illness: developmental handicaps (in children)

JARC—JEWISH ASSOCIATION FOR RESIDENTIAL CARE FOR PERSONS WITH DEVELOPMENTAL DISABILITIES

28366 Franklin Rd.
Southfield, MI 48034
313-352-5272
FAX: 313-352-5279

Type of organization: nonprofit
Public served: individuals/families
Offers: support group(s), housing, food
Disability/chronic illness: developmental disabilities (in Jewish adults)

Comments: A Jewish association that provides residential care and support services to developmentally disabled adults. Operates 13 group homes that provide access to Jewish services, maintains kosher kitchens, and observes Jewish holidays. Although the group primarily services individuals in the Detroit, MI, area, JARC has members nationwide.

JEWISH BRAILLE INSTITUTE OF AMERICA

110 East 30th St.
New York, NY 10016
212-889-2525
FAX: 212-689-3692

Type of organization: nonprofit
Public served: individuals/families, general public, media
Offers: information, reference material, publication(s), research material, products
Disability/chronic illness: visual impairments (in those of Jewish descent)

Comments: Seeks to serve the religious, cultural, educational, and communal needs of the Jewish blind; provides materials in large print, and braille, with large collection in English, Yiddish, Hebrew, and other languages. Has speakers bureau.

JOB ACCOMMODATION NETWORK, WEST VIRGINIA UNIVERSITY

P.O. Box 6080
Morgantown, WV 26506
1-800-526-7234*
304-293-7186
FAX: 304-293-7186

Type of organization: nonprofit, college/university
Public served: individuals/families, general public, media, non-medical professionals, intermediate parties
Offers: information, reference material, counseling, non-medical referrals, rehabilita-

tive services, vocational services

Disability/chronic illness: all

Comments: *In the U.S., except WV. In WV, call 1–800–526–4698. (Both 800 numbers are voice and TDD.) 1–800–DIAL–JAN reaches their electronic bulletin board for the data base. Information and referral service for employers, rehabilitation and social service counselors, and persons with disabilities. Information and counseling service to employers interested in learning how to hire, retain, or promote disabled persons.

JOHN MILTON SOCIETY FOR THE BLIND

475 Riverside Dr., Rm. 455
New York, NY 10115
212–870–3335

Type of organization: nonprofit
Public served: individuals/families
Offers: information, reference material, publication(s), non-medical referrals, financial assistance
Disability/chronic illness: visual impairments

Comments: Provides Christian material (mostly Protestant) for the blind and visually impaired on a worldwide basis. Offers some scholarships and grants to blind students.

JUST ONE BREAK

373 Park Ave. South
New York, NY 10016
212–725–2500
212–725–2046 (TDD)

Type of organization: nonprofit
Public served: individuals/families, intermediate parties
Offers: information, counseling, consultations/guidance, research material, vocational services
Disability/chronic illness: all

Comments: A group of representatives from business, industry, labor, rehabilitation, and medical fields. Active only in New York City. Places qualified handicapped people in competitive employment, offers vocational support services for all applicants, offers testing/evaluation services, public education programs, and more.

JUVENILE DIABETES FOUNDATION

432 Park Ave.
New York, NY 10016
1–800–223–1138
1–800–533–2873

Type of organization: nonprofit
Public served: individuals/families, general public, media, researchers
Offers: information, support group(s), medical referrals, research material
Disability/chronic illness: juvenile diabetes

Comments: Can also be reached at 212–889–7575. Check for local chapters.

K

KESSLER INSTITUTE OF REHABILITATION, PARENTS OF AMPUTEE CHILDREN TOGETHER (PACT)
Pleasant Valley Way
West Orange, NJ 07052
201–731–3600

Type of organization: medical facility
Public served: individuals/families, general public, media
Offers: information, reference material, publication(s), medical referrals, medical services, rehabilitative services
Disability/chronic illness: physical disabilities, amputations

L

LEADER DOGS FOR THE BLIND
1039 South Rochester Rd.
Rochester, MI 48063
313–651–9011
FAX: 313–651–5812

Type of organization: nonprofit
Public served: individuals/families
Offers: education, living aids
Disability/chronic illness: visual impairments

Comments: Provides guide dogs and training for the blind at no charge.

LEARNING HOW
P.O. Box 35481
Charlotte, NC 28235
704–376–4735

Type of organization: nonprofit
Public served: individuals/families
Offers: information, support group(s), counseling, non-medical referrals, seminars/workshops, civil rights assistance/advocacy, vocational services
Disability/chronic illness: all

Comments: Has 19 local groups. Consists of disabled individuals interested in addressing the special needs of members. Strives to build self-esteem and confidence among disabled persons; encourages volunteer community involvement. Seeks to train the disabled for leadership positions and to serve as a support group for disabled persons. Works to prepare members for participation in the job market; acts as a referral service.

LEARNING RESOURCE CENTER

Rehabilitation Institute
of Chicago
345 East Superior St.
Chicago, IL 60611
312–908–2859

Type of organization: medical
facility
Public served: individuals/families,
general public, media, medical
personnel
Offers: information, education,
reference material, consultations/guidance
Disability/chronic illness: physical
disabilities

LITTLE CITY FOUNDATION

4801 West Peterson Ave.,
Ste. 500
Chicago, IL 60646
312–282–2207
FAX: 312–282–0423

Type of organization: nonprofit
Public served: individuals/families
Offers: vocational services,
housing
Disability/chronic illness: mental retardation, emotional disturbance

Comments: Has 3,000 members. Runs a residential community for up to 293 children from six years of age and older. Engages in training, treatment, research, and rehabilitation. Curriculum includes special education and training, an in-cottage training program working in the areas of self-help, self-care, and independent functioning; use of therapy, art therapy, recreational therapy, psychotherapy, and more.

LUPUS FOUNDATION OF AMERICA

1717 Massachusetts Ave. NW,
#203
Washington, DC 20036
1–800–558–0121
202–328–4550

Type of organization: nonprofit
Public served: individuals/families,
general public, media, medical
personnel, researchers
Offers: information, support
group(s), counseling, medical
referrals, research material
Disability/chronic illness: lupus

LUPUS NETWORK
230 Ranch Dr.
Bridgeport, CT 06606
203–372–5795

Type of organization: nonprofit
Public served: individuals/families,
general public, media
Offers: information, reference
material
Disability/chronic illness: lupus,
arthritis

LUTHERAN LIAISON/ NATIONAL CHRISTIAN RESOURCE CENTER
c/o Linda A. Sires
700 Hoffmann Dr.
Watertown, WI 53094
1–800–369–INFO
414–261–3050
FAX: 414–261–8441

Type of organization: nonprofit
Public served: individuals/families,
nonmedical professionals,
intermediate parties
Offers: information, reference
material, publication(s),
consultations/guidance,
seminars/workshops
Disability/chronic illness: mental
retardation

Comments: Has 10 state groups.
Provides information on resources, services, and agencies to
parents, pastors, teachers, advocates, and mental retardation professionals to help them identify
and respond to the physical, social, emotional, and spiritual
needs of persons with mental retardation. Provides habilitation
services for retarded persons, assists in training persons to care for
individuals, and more.

M

MAINSTREAM
3 Bethesda Metro Ctr., Ste. 830
Bethesda, MD 20814
301–654–2400
301–654–2403
FAX: 301–654–2403

Type of organization: nonprofit
Public served: individuals/families,
general public
Offers: information, reference
material, publication(s),
seminars/workshops,
vocational services
Disability/chronic illness: all

Comments: Offers services and
products to increase employment
opportunities. Operates Mainstream Information Network,
which includes a library of books,
periodicals, and directories on
disability-related issues. Also
runs Project LINK (Linking Disabled Individuals with Competi-

62

tive Employment in the Dallas, TX, and Washington, DC, areas).

MARCH OF DIMES BIRTH DEFECT FOUNDATION
1275 Mamaroneck Ave.
White Plains, NY 10605
914-428-7100

Type of organization: nonprofit
Public served: individuals/families, general public, media
Offers: information, education, reference material, publication(s), research material
Disability/chronic illness: birth defects

M.D. ANDERSON HOSPITAL AND TUMOR INSTITUTE RESEARCH MEDICAL LIBRARY
6723 Bertner Ave.
Houston, TX 77030
713-792-2282

Type of organization: medical facility, research facility
Public served: individuals/families, general public, media, medical personnel, nonmedical professionals, researchers
Offers: information, reference material
Disability/chronic illness: cancer

Comments: Open to faculty, students, Texas residents, and visiting scholars.

MEDIC ALERT FOUNDATION INTERNATIONAL
P.O. Box 1009
2323 Colorado Ave.
Turlock, CA 95381
1-800-432-5378*
209-668-3333

Type of organization: nonprofit
Public served: individuals/families, general public, media
Offers: products
Disability/chronic illness: all

Comments: *Other numbers, 1-800-344-3226, 1-800-245-1492. Sells bracelets and/or necklaces with identification number and 800 number individuals can call for more information on the wearer's medical condition in case of an emergency.

MEDICAL CENTER REHABILITATION HOSPITAL, RURAL REHABILITATION TECHNOLOGIES DATABASE (RRTD)
Box 8202, University Station
Grand Forks, ND 58202
701-780-2489

Type of organization: medical facility
Public served: individuals/families, general public, media, medical personnel

Offers: information, publication(s), medical referrals, nonmedical referrals, medical services, products, living aids
Disability/chronic illness: all

Comments: A comprehensive rehabilitation facility that also provides necessary follow-up care and referrals. Also has the Rural Rehabilitation Technologies Database (RRTD) for more information.

MEDICAL MANAGEMENT CONSULTING CORPORATION
106 Quigley Blvd.
New Castle, DE 19720
1–800–654–5438
302–322–0799

Type of organization: private
Public served: individuals/families
Offers: information, nonmedical referrals, products
Disability/chronic illness: diabetes, ostomies, others

Comments: Home medical equipment, including diabetic supplies and ostomy supplies, also provides other 800 numbers for diabetic information.

MENTAL HEALTH INSTITUTE
25 West 81st St.
New York, NY 10024
212–787–7535

Type of organization: nonprofit
Public served: individuals/families
Offers: information, education, diagnostic services, medical referrals, consultations/guidance
Disability/chronic illness: mental illness

MENTAL RETARDATION ASSOCIATION OF AMERICA
221 East 300 South,
Ste. 212
Salt Lake City, UT 84111
801–328–1575

Type of organization: nonprofit
Public served: individuals/families, general public, media, nonmedical professionals, researchers
Offers: information, education, reference material, counseling, civil rights assistance/advocacy, research material, independent living assistance
Disability/chronic illness: mental retardation

Comments: Works to improve the quality of life and advocates for federal programs and financial appropriations for such programs as well as for the rights of the mentally retarded.

MOBILITY INTERNATIONAL U.S.A.
P.O. Box 3551
132 East Broadway
Eugene, OR 97403
503–343–1284
503–343–1284 (TDD)
FAX: 503–343–6812

Type of organization: nonprofit
Public served: individuals/families
Offers: information, reference material, publication(s), non-medical referrals, seminars/workshops, recreational opportunities, travel assistance
Disability/chronic illness: all

Comments: Members include disabled persons, organizations serving the disabled, exchange programs, and libraries. Advocates international, educational, and recreational travel exchange programs that accommodate disabled persons. Provides information on exchange programs, book lists, referrals on homestays with foreign families, and placement in a variety of work-study programs for disabled youths and adults.

MODERN TALKING PICTURES
500 Park St. North
St. Petersburg, FL 33709
813–541–7571

Type of organization: private
Public served: individuals/families
Offers: recreational opportunities, living aids
Disability/chronic illness: hearing impairments

Comments: Offers captioned films and videos. Catalog available.

MONTEFIORE MEDICAL CENTER, HEADACHE UNIT
111 East 210th St.
Bronx, NY 10467
212–920–4636

Type of organization: medical facility, research facility
Public served: individuals/families, general public, media, medical personnel
Offers: information, education, publication(s), medical services, seminars/workshops, research material
Disability/chronic illness: headaches

MOSS REHABILITATION HOSPITAL, TRAVEL INFORMATION SERVICE
1200 West Tabor Rd.
Philadelphia, PA 19141–3099
215–456–9600

Type of organization: nonprofit, medical facility
Public served: individuals/families

Offers: information, travel assistance
Disability/chronic illness: all

Comments: Provides information services for physically disabled travelers on the accessibility of transportation, tourist sites, and accommodations. A division of the Moss Regional Resource and Information Center for Disabled Individuals.

MUSCULAR DYSTROPHY ASSOCIATION
810 7th Ave.
New York, NY 10019
212–586–0808
212–686–6770

Type of organization: nonprofit
Public served: individuals/families, general public, media, medical personnel
Offers: information, education, diagnostic services, reference material, publication(s), medical referrals, research material
Disability/chronic illness: muscular dystrophy

MYASTHENIA GRAVIS FOUNDATION
15 East 26th St.
New York, NY 10010
1–800–541–5454
212–889–8157

Type of organization: nonprofit
Public served: individuals/families, general public, media
Offers: information, medical referrals
Disability/chronic illness: myasthenia gravis

N

NARCOLEPSY AND CATAPLEXY FOUNDATION OF AMERICA
1410 York Ave., Ste. 2D
New York, NY 10021
212–628–6315

Type of organization: nonprofit
Public served: individuals/families, general public, media, medical personnel
Offers: information, education, reference material, publication(s), research material
Disability/chronic illness: narcolepsy, and other sleep disorders

NATIONAL AIDS INFORMATION CLEARINGHOUSE
P.O. Box 6003
Rockville, MD 60003
1–800–458–5231*
301–762–5111

Type of organization: government
Public served: individuals/families, general public, media
Offers: information
Disability/chronic illness: AIDS

Comments: *Call for bulk orders of informational materials.

NATIONAL AMPUTATION FOUNDATION
73 Church St.
Malverne, NY 11565
516–887–3600
FAX: 516–887–3667

Type of organization: nonprofit
Public served: individuals/families
Offers: information, reference material, publication(s), support group(s), counseling, non-medical referrals, rehabilitative services, vocational services
Disability/chronic illness: Amputations

Comments: Assists all amputees in employment, social, and mental rehabilitation. Other services include legal counsel, vocational guidance and placement, social activities, liaison with other groups, and psychological aid. Also, Amp-to-Amp Program and Prosthetic Centre, which makes and repairs prosthetic devices as well as trains individuals to use them.

NATIONAL AMPUTEE GOLF ASSOCIATION
P.O. Box 1228
Amherst, NH 03031
1–800–633–6242
603–673–1135

Type of organization: nonprofit
Public served: individuals/families
Offers: information, reference material, publication(s), recreational opportunities
Disability/chronic illness: amputation of hand or foot or combination

Comments: Promotes golf for amputees; sponsors local, regional, national, and international tournaments as well as "first swing" program for therapists. Data base of address listings and demographic information.

NATIONAL ASSOCIATION OF ATOMIC VETERANS
P.O. Box 4424
Salem, MA 01970
1–800–955–1186
508–744–9396
FAX: 508–740–9267

Type of organization: nonprofit
Public served: individuals/families
Offers: information, reference material, publication(s), support group(s), civil rights assistance/advocacy

Disability/chronic illness: exposure to (military-related) atomic radiation

Comments: Aids with service-connected disability claims for those exposed to atomic radiation (tests as well as Nagasaki/Hiroshima occupation forces). Participates in related legislative activities.

NATIONAL ASSOCIATION OF THE DEAF

814 Thayer Ave.
Silver Spring, MD 20910
301–587–1788
301–587–1789 (TDD)
FAX: 301–587–1791

Type of organization: nonprofit
Public served: individuals/families
Offers: information, publication(s), support group(s), counseling
Disability/chronic illness: hearing impairments

NATIONAL ASSOCIATION FOR INDEPENDENT LIVING, INDEPENDENT ASSOCIATION

55 City Hall Plaza
Brockton, MA 02401
508–559–9091
FAX: 508–580–4345

Type of organization: nonprofit
Public served: individuals/families, general public, media

Offers: information, publication(s), support group(s), nonmedical referrals, seminars/workshops, civil rights assistance/advocacy, independent living assistance
Disability/chronic illness: all

Comments: A division of National Rehabilitation Association. Seeks to promote independent living, works to remove barriers, create new options, and provide support services that will enable persons with disabilities to control their own lives.

NATIONAL ASSOCIATION FOR PARENTS OF VISUALLY IMPAIRED, INC.

2180 Linway
Beloit, WI 53511
1–800–562–6265
608–362–4945

Type of organization: nonprofit
Public served: individuals/families, general public, media, nonmedical professionals
Offers: information, reference material, publication(s), support group(s), counseling, nonmedical referrals, research material
Disability/chronic illness: visual impairments (in children)

Comments: Seeks to provide support to families of the visually impaired child. Also open to community groups and interested individuals. Provides information on services, education, and treatment for the children. Another goal is to increase public awareness of the visually impaired.

NATIONAL ASSOCIATION OF THE PHYSICALLY HANDICAPPED

Bethesda Scarlet Oaks,
No. GA4
440 Lafayette Ave.
Cincinnati, OH 45220-1000
513-961-8040

Type of organization: nonprofit
Public served: individuals/families
Offers: information, publication(s), support group(s), civil rights assistance/advocacy
Disability/chronic illness: physical disabilities

Comments: Members are physically handicapped. Group seeks to involve disabled persons in the planning and administration of all programs in their interest. Seeks to advance the social, economic, and physical welfare of the physically handicapped.

NATIONAL ASSOCIATION OF PRIVATE RESIDENTIAL RESOURCES

4200 Evergreen Ln., #315
Anandale, VA 22003
703-642-6614

Type of organization: nonprofit
Public served: individuals/families, media
Offers: information, reference material, publication(s), civil rights assistance/advocacy, independent living assistance
Disability/chronic illness: developmental disabilities

Comments: Primarily a coalition of agencies that serve the developmentally disabled but includes some others interested in the field of private residential services. Committed to enhancing the quality of life for persons along with a direct concern for all living situations. Works with others to provide services necessary for fulfillment of other human needs.

NATIONAL ASSOCIATION OF PSYCHIATRIC SURVIVORS (NAPS)

P.O. Box 618
Sioux Falls, SD 57101
605-334-4067

Type of organization: nonprofit
Public served: individuals/families, general public, media
Offers: information, reference material, publication(s), support group(s), nonmedical referrals, civil rights assistance/advocacy
Disability/chronic illness: mental illness

Comments: Has local groups. Seeks to promote the rights of psychiatric patients and end what the group identifies as involuntary psychiatric intervention, including civil commitment and forced treatments like electroshock, psychosurgery, involuntary detention, and mood-altering drug therapies. Encourages development of voluntary alternatives, including self-help and peer support groups and other nonmedical treatments. Promotes freedom of choice for individuals in selecting mental treatments and the right to refuse any unwanted treatments. Challenges negative social attitudes regarding mental illness and promotes public understanding and sensitivity for people who have received psychiatric treatment.

NATIONAL ASSOCIATION FOR VISUALLY HANDICAPPED
22 West 21st St.
New York, NY 10010
212–889–3141
FAX: 212–727–2931

Type of organization: nonprofit
Public served: individuals/families, general public, media, nonmedical professionals
Offers: information, reference material, support group(s), counseling, recreational opportunities, products
Disability/chronic illness: visual impairments

Comments: Source for large-print textbooks, pleasure-reading books for partially sighted. A clearinghouse for more information. Association includes foundations, agencies, organizations, clubs, and individuals.

NATIONAL ASTHMA CENTER LUNG LINE INFORMATION SERVICE
National Jewish Hospital/
    National Asthma Center
3800 East Colfax Ave.
Denver, CO 80206
1–800–222–5864 (in U.S.,
    except CO)
303–398–1477

Type of organization: medical
facility
Public served: individuals/families,
general public, media
Offers: information, counseling,
medical referrals
Disability/chronic illness: asthma

Comments: Call 303–355–LUNG
to reach an automated phone line.

NATIONAL BRAILLE PRESS
88 Stephen St.
Boston, MA 02115
617–266–6160
FAX: 617–437–0456

Type of organization: nonprofit
Public served: individuals/families
Offers: publication(s), recre-
ational opportunities
Disability/chronic illness: visual
impairments

Comments: Publishes large-type
books, books in braille; does contract printing for organizations.
Sponsors the Children's Braille
Book Club. Publishes a newsletter, *National Braille Press Re-
lease,* twice a year and a monthly
magazine, *Our Special,* in braille.

NATIONAL CENTER FOR DISABILITY SERVICES
201 I.U. Willets Rd.
Albertson, NY 11507
516–747–5400
FAX: 516–747–5378

Type of organization: nonprofit
Public served: individuals/families,
general public, media
Offers: information, diagnostic
services, reference material,
publication(s), counseling,
medical referrals, nonmedical
referrals, medical services,
consultations/guidance, sem-
inars/workshops, research
material, rehabilitative services, vocational services
Disability/chronic illness: all

Comments: Provides educational,
vocational, rehabilitation, and research opportunities for persons
with disabilities. Has: Abilities
Health and Rehabilitation Services,
Career Employment Institute, Research and Training Institute, and
Henry Viscardi School.

NATIONAL CENTER ON EMPLOYMENT OF THE DEAF
National Technical Institute
for the Deaf
One Lomb Memorial Drive
Rochester, NY 14623
716–475–6834
716–475–6205 (TDD)

Type of organization: nonprofit
Public served: individuals/families
Offers: information, vocational
services
Disability/chronic illness: hearing
impairments

NATIONAL CENTER FOR THERAPEUTIC RIDING

Rock Creek Park Horse Ctr.
P.O. Box 42501
Washington, DC 20015
202–966–8004
FAX: 202–686–3454

Type of organization: nonprofit
Public served: individuals/families, nonmedical professionals
Offers: information, recreational opportunities
Disability/chronic illness: all

Comments: Specialized riding programs for the physically handicapped, emotionally disturbed, learning disabled, and mentally retarded. Open to those in the Washington, DC, area.

NATIONAL CENTER FOR YOUTH WITH DISABILITIES

University of Minnesota
420 Delaware St. SE
P.O. Box 721
Minneapolis, MN 55455
1–800–333–6293
612–626–2825*
FAX: 612–626–2134

Type of organization: nonprofit, college/university
Public served: individuals/families, general public, media, medical personnel, nonmedical professionals, intermediate parties
Offers: information, education, reference material, publication(s), consultations/guidance
Disability/chronic illness: all

Comments: *612–624–3939 (TDD). An adolescent health program. Computer-accessible database for youth-related information on chronic or disabling conditions. Seeks to enable adolescents and young adults with chronic illnesses or developmental disabilities to participate in community life to their fullest capacity. Fosters cooperation among agencies, professionals, parents, and youth.

NATIONAL CHRONIC PAIN OUTREACH ASSOCIATION

7979 Old Georgetown Rd.
Bethesda, MD 20814
301–652–4948
FAX: 301–907–0745

Type of organization: nonprofit
Public served: individuals/families, general public, media
Offers: information, support group(s), counseling, medical referrals
Disability/chronic illness: chronic pain

Comments: Serves as a clearing-house for information about chronic pain and its management. Publishes a quarterly newsletter, *Lifeline,* and offers audiocassettes on a wide range of pain management topics. Provides information on starting new support groups. Has local chapters nationwide.

NATIONAL COUNCIL ON INDEPENDENT LIVING (NCIL)
Troy Atrium
4th St. and Broadway
Troy, NY 12180
518-274-1979
FAX: 518-841-6168

Type of organization: nonprofit
Public served: individuals/families, intermediate parties
Offers: information, reference material, publication(s), support group(s), counseling, non-medical referrals, seminars/ workshops, independent living assistance
Disability/chronic illness: all

Comments: *Can also be reached at 518-491-9013 (computer network) or 518-848-3101 (TDD). 80 local groups and 380 members, which includes independent living centers, organizations that provide support to independent living centers, and individuals.

NATIONAL DEAF BOWLING ASSOCIATION
9244 East Mansfield Ave.
Denver, CO 80237
303-771-9018

Type of organization: nonprofit
Public served: individuals/families, general public
Offers: recreational opportunities
Disability/chronic illness: hearing impairments

Comments: 20 local groups. Individuals, clubs, and organizations of hearing-impaired bowlers. Conducts bowling tournaments, including the World's Deaf Bowling Championship, National Deaf Team Doubles-Singles, and National Deaf Master Tournament.

NATIONAL DEAF WOMEN'S BOWLING ASSOCIATION
c/o Kathy M. Darby
33 August Rd.
Simsbury, CT 06070
203-651-8234

Type of organization: nonprofit
Public served: individuals/families

Offers: recreational opportunities
Disability/chronic illness: hearing
  impairments (in women)

Comments: Hearing-impaired
bowlers. Promotes fellowship and
fair play among participants. Annual tournaments with singles,
doubles, team, queen's, and world
championship.

NATIONAL DOWN
SYNDROME CONGRESS
1800 Dempster St.
Park Ridge, IL 60068–1146
1–800–232–6372
708–823–7550
FAX: 708–823–9528

Type of organization: nonprofit
Public served: individuals/families,
  general public, media
Offers: information, publica-
  tion(s), support group(s),
  counseling, medical referrals,
  nonmedical referrals, civil
  rights assistance/advocacy
Disability/chronic illness: Down
  syndrome

Comments: Families of individuals
with Down syndrome, educators,
health professionals, and other interested individuals who wish to
promote the welfare of these individuals. Promotes the belief that
they have the right to a normal and
dignified life, particularly in the
areas of education, medical care,
employment, and human services.
Has local groups.

NATIONAL DOWN
SYNDROME SOCIETY
666 Broadway
New York, NY 10012
1–800–221–4602
212–460–9330
FAX: 212–979–2873

Type of organization: nonprofit
Public served: individuals/families,
  general public, media, medical
  personnel, nonmedical
  professionals
Offers: information, publica-
  tion(s), support group(s),
  counseling, medical referrals,
  nonmedical referrals, sem-
  inars/workshops, civil rights
  assistance/advocacy, research
  material
Disability/chronic illness: Down's
  syndrome

Comments: Works to increase public awareness, supports research
into cause and treatment, information and referral, educational
programs, directory of parent
support groups and early intervention programs.

NATIONAL EASTER SEAL SOCIETY FOR CRIPPLED CHILDREN AND ADULTS
70 East Lake St.
Chicago, IL 60601
312-726-6200
312-726-4258 (TDD)
FAX: 312-726-1494

Type of organization: nonprofit
Public served: individuals/families, general public, media, medical personnel, nonmedical professionals, intermediate parties
Offers: information, education, reference material, publication(s), support group(s), counseling, medical referrals, nonmedical referrals, recreational opportunities, civil rights assistance/advocacy, research material, rehabilitative services
Disability/chronic illness: physical disabilities

Comments: 67 state groups and 98 local groups. Federation of state and local societies that operate over 400 service centers. Seeks to establish and conduct programs for people with disabilities; works with other groups and agencies to provide needed services to disabled.

NATIONAL FEDERATION OF THE BLIND
1800 Johnson St.
Baltimore, MD 21230
1-800-638-7518*
410-659-9314
FAX: 410-685-5653

Type of organization: nonprofit
Public served: individuals/families, general public, media
Offers: information, reference material, publication(s), medical referrals, seminars/workshops, financial assistance, civil rights assistance/advocacy, research material
Disability/chronic illness: visual impairments

Comments: *Job opportunity number. 50 state and 600 local organizations. Seeks to promote equality and integration of blind into society. Provides scholarships, promotes research and public awareness. Monitors legislative issues, legal cases, and social concerns.

NATIONAL FOUNDATION FOR ASTHMA
P.O. Box 30069
Tucson, AZ 85751-0069
602-323-6046

Type of organization: medical
facility
Public served: individuals/families,
general public, media
Offers: information, education,
publication(s), medical
services
Disability/chronic illness: asthma

NATIONAL FOUNDATION FOR CHILDREN'S HEARING, EDUCATION AND RESEARCH

928 McLean Ave.
Yonkers, NY 10704
914–633–1505

Type of organization: research
facility
Public served: individuals/families,
general public, media
Offers: information, publica-
tion(s), financial assistance,
research material
Disability/chronic illness: hearing
impairments

Comments: Has speech and hearing center in Yonkers.

NATIONAL FOUNDATION FOR FIBROMYALGIA

P.O. Box 3429
San Diego, CA 92163–1429
1–800–251–9528
619–291–8649
FAX: 619–574–1101

Type of organization: nonprofit
Public served: individuals/families,
general public, media, medical
personnel, nonmedical
professionals
Offers: information, education,
reference material, publica-
tion(s), support group(s),
counseling, medical referrals,
nonmedical referrals, consul-
tations/guidance, seminars/
workshops, research
material
Disability/chronic illness: fibromyalgia

Comments: Association of local
support groups, state fibromyalgia organizations, and others interested in fibromyalgia.

NATIONAL FOUNDATION FOR HAPPY HORSEMANSHIP FOR THE HANDICAPPED

P.O. Box 462
Malvern, PA 19355
215–644–7414

Type of organization: nonprofit,
professional
Public served: individuals/families
Offers: information, education,
reference material, seminars/
workshops, recreational
opportunities, vocational
services
Disability/chronic illness: all

Comments: A group of individuals who assist handicapped persons in their involvement with horses as a form of therapy and rehabilitation. Purpose is to encourage and unify the teaching of the disabled to ride or drive horses through training of personnel and exchange among those who have experience in the field. Provides films and sponsors how-to clinics for volunteers. Maintains speakers bureau and library.

NATIONAL FOUNDATION OF WHEELCHAIR TENNIS
940 Calle Amanecer, Ste. B
San Clemente, CA 92672
714–361–6811
FAX: 714–361–6822

Type of organization: nonprofit
Public served: individuals/families
Offers: information, reference material, publication(s), seminars/workshops, recreational opportunities
Disability/chronic illness: physical disabilities

Comments: Organizes, promotes, and encourages participation in tennis for those with an orthopedic disability. Offers training to schools, parks and recreation programs, tennis professionals, and others. Holds Junior Wheelchair Sports Camp program for disabled children from 7 to 18 years of age.

NATIONAL FRAGILE X SYNDROME SUPPORT GROUP
RR 8, Box 109
Bridgeton, NJ 08302
609–455–7508

Type of organization: nonprofit
Public served: individuals/families, general public, media, medical personnel
Offers: information, reference material, support group(s), medical referrals
Disability/chronic illness: fragile x syndrome

NATIONAL HANDICAPPED SPORTS
451 Hungerford Dr., Ste. 100
Rockville, MD 20850
1–800–966–4NHS
301–217–0960*
FAX: 301–217–0968

Type of organization: nonprofit
Public served: individuals/families
Offers: information, education, recreational opportunities
Disability/chronic illness: any mobility impairment for any reason, from spinal cord injury to amputation, or visual impairment

Comments: *301–217–0963 (TDD). Promotes sports and recreation opportunities, including winter and summer programs in skiing, sailing, racing, competitive alpine and nordic skiing, archery, basketball, cycling, lawnbowling, shooting, swimming, table tennis, track and field, volleyball, and weight-lifting, with special programs for children, women, and veterans.

NATIONAL HEARING ASSOCIATION
721 Enterprise Dr.
Oak Brook, IL 60521
312–323–7200

Type of organization: nonprofit
Public served: individuals/families, general public, media, medical personnel
Offers: information, reference materials, consultations/ guidance, seminars/ workshops
Disability/chronic illness: hearing impairments

NATIONAL HEMOPHILIA FOUNDATION
19 West 34th St., Ste. 1204
New York, NY 10001
212–563–0211

Type of organization: medical facility, research facility
Public served: individuals/families, general public, media, medical personnel, researchers
Offers: information, education, reference material, medical referrals, medical services, consultations/guidance, research material
Disability/chronic illness: hemophilia, blood disorders

NATIONAL INDUSTRIES FOR THE BLIND
524 Hamburg Turnpike, CN 969
Wayne, NJ 07470–0969
201–595–9200
FAX: 201–595–9122

Type of organization: nonprofit
Public served: individuals/families
Offers: vocational services
Disability/chronic illness: visual impairments

Comments: Represents 110 workshops that employ the blind to fulfill contracts to the federal government. Open to those individuals who are able and wish to work. Located in 37 states, Puerto Rico, and Washington, DC. The association researches new products and provides such services as management, quality control, and engineering to increase the efficiency and broaden the job opportunities.

NATIONAL INFORMATION CENTER FOR CHILDREN AND YOUTH WITH DISABILITIES (NICHCY)
P.O. Box 1492
Washington, DC 20013
1-800-999-5599
703-893-6061*

Type of organization: nonprofit
Public served: individuals/families, general public, media, medical personnel, nonmedical professionals
Offers: information, reference material, publication(s), non-medical referrals
Disability/chronic illness: all

Comments: *703-843-8614 (TDD). Clearinghouse for information. Provides information to parents, educators, care-givers, advocates, and others to help children and youth with disabilities become active members of their communities. Provides personal responses to specific questions and technical assistance to parent and professional groups. Also maintains library.

NATIONAL INFORMATION CLEARINGHOUSE FOR INFANTS WITH DISABILITIES AND LIFE-THREATENING CONDITIONS
Benson Bldg., 1st Fl.
Columbia, SC 29208
1-800-922-9234
1-800-922-1107 (in SC)

Type of organization: college/university
Public served: individuals/families, medical personnel
Offers: information, support group(s), counseling, medical referrals, financial assistance, civil rights assistance/advocacy
Disability/chronic illness: all

NATIONAL INSTITUTE FOR REHABILITATION ENGINEERING
P.O. Box T
Hewitt, NJ 07421
1-800-736-2216
201-853-6585

Type of organization: nonprofit, research facility
Public served: individuals/families
Offers: information, research material, products, living aids, independent living assistance
Disability/chronic illness: severe physical disabilities, multiple disabilities

Comments: Multidisciplinary research, training, and service organization that provides custom-designed and custom-made tools and devices along with intensive personal task-performance and driver training to help the handicapped become more self-sufficient and independent. Sometimes considered the "last resort" for help in these situations.

NATIONAL KIDNEY FOUNDATION
2 Park Ave.
New York, NY 10016
1-800-622-9010
212-889-2210

Type of organization: nonprofit
Public served: individuals/families, general public, media
Offers: information, support group(s), counseling, recreational opportunities, research material
Disability/chronic illness: kidney diseases

Comments: Local chapters nationwide.

NATIONAL LEUKEMIA ASSOCIATION
Lower Concourse, Roosevelt Field
Garden City, NY 11530
516-741-1190

Type of organization: nonprofit
Public served: individuals/families
Offers: financial assistance, research material
Disability/chronic illness: leukemia

Comments: Provides financial aid for treatment of leukemia.

NATIONAL LUPUS ERYTHEMATOSUS FOUNDATION
5430 Van Nuys Blvd., Ste. 206
Van Nuys, CA 91401
818-885-8787

Type of organization: nonprofit
Public served: individuals/families, general public, media, medical personnel
Offers: information, reference material, publication(s), counseling, seminars/workshops, research material
Disability/chronic illness: lupus

NATIONAL MARFAN FOUNDATION
54 Irma Ave.
Port Washington, NY 11050
1-800-862-7326
516-883-8712

Type of organization: nonprofit
Public served: individuals/families, general public, media, medical personnel

Offers: information, support group(s), research material
Disability/chronic illness: Marfan syndrome, arthritis

NATIONAL MENTAL HEALTH ASSOCIATION
1021 Prince St.
Alexandria, VA 22314
1–800–969–6642
703–684–7722
FAX: 703–684–5968

Type of organization: nonprofit
Public served: individuals/families, general public, media
Offers: information, medical referrals
Disability/chronic illness: mental illness

NATIONAL MENTAL HEALTH CONSUMER SELF-HELP CLEARINGHOUSE
311 South Juniper St., Rm. 902
Philadelphia, PA 19107
1–800–688–4226
215–735–6367

Type of organization: nonprofit
Public served: individuals/families
Offers: information, publication(s), support group(s), nonmedical referrals, consultations/guidance
Disability/chronic illness: mental illness

Comments: Serves mental health consumers/ex-patients and consumer/ex-patient self-help groups. Provides technical assistance in the development of self-help projects. Offers informational referrals, written material, and consulting services. Has 300 groups. Data base of technical assistance providers.

NATIONAL MIGRAINE FOUNDATION
777 7th Ave.
New York, NY 10019
212–247–4000*

Type of organization: nonprofit
Public served: individuals/families, general public, media, medical personnel
Offers: information, reference material, publication(s), medical referrals, consultations/guidance, seminars/workshops, research material
Disability/chronic illness: migraine headaches

Comments: *Ask for extension M-62.

NATIONAL MULTIPLE SCLEROSIS SOCIETY
205 East 42nd St.
New York, NY 10017
1–800–624–8236
212–986–3240

Type of organization: nonprofit
Public served: individuals/families, general public, media, medical personnel, researchers
Offers: information, support group(s), counseling, medical referrals, recreational opportunities, research material
Disability/chronic illness: multiple sclerosis

Comments: Local chapters nationwide.

NATIONAL OCEAN ACCESS PROJECT
Annapolis City Marina
P.O. Box 3377
Annapolis, MD 21403
410–280–0464

Type of organization: nonprofit
Public served: individuals/families, general public
Offers: information, publication(s), nonmedical referrals, recreational opportunities
Disability/chronic illness: all

Comments: 500 members. Develops and promotes marine recreational opportunities for people with disabilities. Provides referrals and technical assistance in fishing, kayaking, power boating, rowing, sailing, scuba diving, and water skiing. Offers Learn-to-Sail programs. Sponsors annual Independence Cup regatta for sailors with disabilities. Conducts model boat races, maintains speakers bureau.

NATIONAL ODD SHOE EXCHANGE
7102 North 35th Ave., Ste. 2
Phoenix, AZ 85051
602–841–6691
FAX: 602–841–3349

Type of organization: nonprofit
Public served: individuals/families
Offers: information
Disability/chronic illness: amputations of or differences in hands or feet due to birth defect, accident, disease, or injury

Comments: A shoe exchange that seeks to link those with mutual shoe problems in order to swap shoes they have and can't use or will not need in the future. Maintains National Odd Shoe Foundation, National Odd Shoe Store and catalogs. Also operates an odd glove exchange.

NATIONAL ORGANIZATION FOR RARE DISORDERS
Fairwood Professional Bldg. 100
Rt. 37, Box K
New Fairfield, CT 06812
1–800–447–NORD
203–746–6518

Type of organization: nonprofit
Public served: individuals/families, general public, researchers
Offers: information, research material
Disability/chronic illness: rare disorders

Comments: Coalition of health organizations that deal with rare disorders.

NATIONAL ORGANIZATION ON DISABILITY

910 16th St. NW, Ste. 600
Washington, DC 20006
1–800–248–2253
202–293–5960
FAX: 202–293–7999

Type of organization: nonprofit
Public served: individuals/families, general public, media
Offers: information, reference material, publication(s), seminars/workshops, recreational opportunities, civil rights assistance/advocacy
Disability/chronic illness: all

Comments: Works to improve public image of disabled, to involve disabled and others in voluntary working partnerships, and to promote greater educational and employment opportunities, improve access to buildings, polling places, and transportation, increase participation in recreational, social, religious, electoral, and cultural activities.

NATIONAL OSTEOPOROSIS FOUNDATION

1150 17th St. NW, #500
Washington, DC 20036
1–800–223–9994
202–223–2226
FAX: 202–223–2237

Type of organization: nonprofit
Public served: individuals/families, general public, media, medical personnel, researchers
Offers: information
Disability/chronic illness: osteoporosis

Comments: Dedicated to finding answers to help women overcome the disease. Members receive information about preventing and treating osteoporosis. Publishes quarterly newsletter.

NATIONAL PARAPLEGIA FOUNDATION

333 North Michigan Ave.
Chicago, IL 60601
312–346–4779

Type of organization: nonprofit
Public served: individuals/families
Offers: nonmedical referrals, rehabilitative services, vocational services

Disability/chronic illness: spinal cord injuries

Comments: Job referral services are provided.

NATIONAL PARENT CHAIN
Coalition for Handicapped
   Americans Information
   Network
867-C High St.
Worthington, OH 43805
614–431–1911

Type of organization: nonprofit
Public served: individuals/families, general public, medical personnel, nonmedical professionals
Offers: information
Disability/chronic illness: all

Comments: National information and education network that links existing coalitions and organizations, as well as consumers with state and federal governments.

NATIONAL PARKINSON'S FOUNDATION
University of Miami
   School of Medicine
1501 Northwest 9th Ave.
Miami, FL 33136
1–800–327–4545
1–800–433–7022 (in FL)*

Type of organization: nonprofit, college/university

Public served: individuals/families, general public, media, researchers
Offers: information, medical services, research material, rehabilitative services
Disability/chronic illness: Parkinson's disease

Comments: *In Miami, call 305–547–6666.

NATIONAL SCOLIOSIS FOUNDATION
P.O. Box 547
Belmont, MA 02178
617–489–0888

Type of organization: nonprofit
Public served: individuals/families, general public, media
Offers: information, reference material, publication(s)
Disability/chronic illness: scoliosis, spinal cord abnormalities

NATIONAL SOCIETY TO PREVENT BLINDNESS
500 East Remington Rd.
Schaumburg, IL 60173
1–800–331–2020
708–843–2020
FAX: 708–843–8458

Type of organization: nonprofit, professional
Public served: individuals/families, general public, medical per-

sonnel, nonmedical professionals

Offers: information, education, diagnostic services, reference material, publication(s), counseling, seminars/workshops, research material, living aids

Disability/chronic illness: visual impairments

Comments: Open to both professionals and laypeople who are interested in preventing blindness and conserving eyesight. Promotes research, public education, glaucoma and preschool vision testing. Has 3,000-volume library.

NATIONAL SPINAL CORD INJURY ASSOCIATION

600 West Cummings,
  Ste. 2000
Woburn, MA 01801
1-800-962-9629 (in U.S.,
  except MA)
617-935-2722

Type of organization: nonprofit
Public served: individuals/families, general public, media
Offers: information, research material, rehabilitative services
Disability/chronic illness: spinal cord injuries

Comments: Also sponsors In Touch with Kids, a network for parents of children with spinal cord injury or disease.

NATIONAL STROKE ASSOCIATION

300 Hampden Ave., Ste. 240
Englewood, CO 80110
303-839-1992

Type of organization: nonprofit
Public served: individuals/families, general public, media, medical personnel
Offers: information, reference material, publication(s), support group(s), medical referrals, nonmedical referrals
Disability/chronic illness: stroke

NATIONAL TAY-SACHS AND ALLIED DISEASES ASSOCIATION

92 Washington Ave.
Cedarhurst, NY 11516
516-569-4300

Type of organization: nonprofit
Public served: individuals/families, general public, media, medical personnel
Offers: information, reference material, publication(s), medical referrals, research material
Disability/chronic illness: Tay-Sachs disease

NATIONAL WHEELCHAIR ATHLETIC ASSOCIATION

3595 East Fountain Blvd.,
    Ste. L-1
Colorado Springs, CO 80910
719–574–1150
719–574–9840

Type of organization: nonprofit
Public served: individuals/families
Offers: information, publication(s), recreational opportunities
Disability/chronic illness: physical disabilities in conjunction with significant permanent neuromuscular-skeletal disability

Comments: Members are men and women in wheelchairs who compete in various amateur sports events, such as track and field, swimming, archery, shooting, table tennis, and weightlifting. Competitions held on the regional level and then on the national level to select representatives for the U.S. in international competitions.

NATIONAL WHEELCHAIR BASKETBALL ASSOCIATION

University of Kentucky
110 Seaton Bldg.
Lexington, KY 40506–0219
606–257–1623

Type of organization: nonprofit
Public served: individuals/families, general public, media
Offers: information, publication(s), recreational opportunities
Disability/chronic illness: physical disabilities of the lower extremities

Comments: 28 conferences. Wheelchair basketball teams are comprised of individuals with severe permanent physical disabilities. Seeks to provide opportunities on a national basis for the physically disabled to participate in the sport of wheelchair basketball, with its adjunct psychological, social, and emotional benefits, and to maintain a high level of competition. Sponsors sectional and regional tournaments.

NATIONAL WHEELCHAIR SOFTBALL ASSOCIATION

1616 Todd Ct.
Hastings, MN 55033
612–437–1792

Type of organization: nonprofit
Public served: individuals/families
Offers: information, seminars/workshops, recreational opportunities
Disability/chronic illness: physical disabilities

Comments: Teams of wheelchair softball players. Sponsors tournaments, holds training seminars, and acts as governing body for the promotion, interpretation, standardization, and growth of wheelchair softball.

NETWORKING PROJECT FOR DISABLED WOMEN AND GIRLS

c/o YWCA of City of New York
610 Lexington Ave.
New York, NY 10022
212-735-9767

Type of organization: nonprofit
Public served: individuals/families
Offers: information, support group(s), counseling, consultations/guidance, civil rights assistance/advocacy, vocational services
Disability/chronic illness: all

Comments: Seeks to connect adolescent girls who have disabilities with adult women role models who also have disabilities. Offers advocacy training, pre-employment skills development, and one-to-one mentoring. This project operates only in New York but the group provides advice for those who are interested in establishing similar programs in other cities.

NEUROTICS ANONYMOUS INTERNATIONAL LIAISON

11140 Bainbridge Dr.
Little Rock, AR 72212
501-221-2809

Type of organization: nonprofit
Public served: individuals/families
Offers: support group(s), counseling
Disability/chronic illness: mental illness, neuroses

Comments: 10,000 members. Consists of individuals suffering or recovering from emotional illnesses who use the techniques of Neurotics Anonymous to aid and maintain their recovery. Organization has adapted the Twelve Steps of Alcoholics Anonymous World Services and applied them to the problems of mentally and emotionally disturbed (neurotic) individuals. Members exchange and discuss experiences and recovery stories.

NISH (NATIONAL INDUSTRIES FOR THE SEVERELY HANDICAPPED

2235 Cedar Ln.
Vienna, VA 22182-5200
703-560-6800

Type of organization: nonprofit
Public served: individuals/families,
intermediate parties
Offers: information, publi-
cation(s), consultations/
guidance, vocational services
Disability/chronic illness: severe
handicaps

Comments: Provides employment
opportunities for people with severe disabilities under the Javits-
Wagner O'Day Act. Promotes
their placement in competitive in-
dustries. Conducts research and
development to identify for the
government commodities and services that are feasible for work
centers. Provides training and
technical assistance to those centers.

NORTH AMERICAN RIDING FOR THE HANDICAPPED ASSOCIATION
P.O. Box 33150
Denver, CO 80233
1–800–369–7433
303–452–1212
FAX: 303–252–4610

Type of organization: nonprofit
Public served: individuals/families,
nonmedical professionals
Offers: information, recreational
opportunities
Disability/chronic illness: all

Comments: Open to both individuals and centers devoted to therapeutic riding for disabled persons.
Offers training and certification
for instructors.

O

OBSESSIVE-COMPULSIVE ANONYMOUS
P.O. Box 215
New Hyde Park, NY 11040
516–741–4901
FAX: 212–768–4679

Type of organization: nonprofit
Public served: individuals/families
Offers: support group(s)
Disability/chronic illness: mental
illness

Comments: 45 regional groups.
For individuals suffering from
obsessive-compulsive disorders.
Follows the twelve-step method
established by Alcoholics Anonymous World Services.

ONE-ARM DOVE HUNT ASSOCIATION
Box 582
Olney, TX 76374
817–564–2102

Type of organization: nonprofit
Public served: individuals/families
Offers: information, recreational
opportunities

Disability/chronic illness: amputation of hand or arm

Comments: Amputees who enjoy the sport of shotgun shooting; also interested nonamputees. Purpose is to help amputees accept their handicap and to provide fellowship and shooting competitions. Activities include dove hunts, One-Arm Tales, One-Arm Talent, and dove dinners. Bestows awards.

ONE TO ONE
One World Trade Center, 105th Fl.
New York, NY 10048
212–938–5300

Type of organization: nonprofit
Public served: individuals/families, general public, media
Offers: information, reference material, support group(s), civil rights assistance/ advocacy
Disability/chronic illness: mental retardation

Comments: A mentoring program.

ONE SHOE CREW, THE
86 Clavela Ave.
Sacramento, CA 95828
916–364–SHOE

Type of organization: nonprofit
Public served: individuals/families

Offers: publication(s), products
Disability/chronic illness: amputation, others who have lost a foot

Comments: A service organization that finds cost-sharing partners for people who wear only one shoe or those who wear two mismated shoes. Matches shoe size and width of clients seeking partners. Over 35,000 new, unused shoes are available at no cost. Client must prepay shipping. Clients indicate the general shoe style they prefer and receive pictures of what is available in their size and width.

P

PAGET'S DISEASE FOUNDATION
P.O. Box 2772
Brooklyn, NY 11202
718–596–1043

Type of organization: nonprofit
Public served: individuals/families, general public, media, medical personnel
Offers: information, publication(s), medical referrals, consultations/guidance, research material
Disability/chronic illness: Paget's disease

PAIN MANAGEMENT CENTER
Department of Psychiatry,
  Mayo Foundation
200 First St. SW
Rochester, MN 55901
507–284–2933

Type of organization: medical
  facility, research facility
Public served: individuals/families
Offers: information, counseling,
  medical services, seminars/
  workshops, research material
Disability/chronic illness: chronic
  pain

PAIN TREATMENT CENTER
622 West 168th St.
New York, NY 10032
212–694–7114

Type of organization: medical
  facility, research facility
Public served: individuals/families,
  medical personnel
Offers: information, diagnostic
  services, medical referrals,
  medical services, consul-
  tations/guidance, research
  material
Disability/chronic illness: chronic
  pain

Comments: By physician referral
only.

PARA-AMPS
P.O. Box 515
South Beloit, IL 61080
608–362–3627

Type of organization: nonprofit
Public served: individuals/families
Offers: support group(s)
Disability/chronic illness: all

Comments: Pen pal program for
gay handicapped individuals. Offers medical, financial, and
support-group information.

PARENTS OF DOWN SYNDROME CHILDREN
c/o Montgomery County
  Association for Retarded
  Citizens
11600 Nebel St.
Rockville, MD 20852
301–984–5792

Type of organization: nonprofit
Public served: individuals/families
Offers: information, publica-
  tion(s), support group(s),
  counseling, medical referrals,
  nonmedical referrals
Disability/chronic illness: Down
  syndrome

Comments: Primarily a local support system for parents and families.

90

PARKINSON'S EDUCATIONAL PROGRAM
1800 Park Newport, Ste. 302
Newport Beach, CA 92660
1-800-344-7872
714-640-0218

Type of organization: nonprofit
Public served: individuals/families, general public, media, medical personnel, researchers
Offers: information, support group(s), counseling, medical referrals, civil rights assistance/advocacy, research material
Disability/chronic illness: Parkinson's disease, central nervous system injury and disease

PAWS WITH A CAUSE
1235 100th St. SE
Byron Center, MI 49315
616-698-0688
616-698-0688 (TDD)
FAX: 616-698-2988

Type of organization: nonprofit
Public served: individuals/families, nonmedical professionals
Offers: information, products, living aids
Disability/chronic illness: any that cause need for a service dog

Comments: Trains and provides dogs to assist people with disabilities. Works to increase awareness of the need for service dogs and legal access rights. Conducts educational programs.

PILOT GUIDE DOG FOUNDATION
625 West Town St.
Columbus, OH 43215
614-221-6367

Type of organization: nonprofit
Public served: individuals/families
Offers: living aids
Disability/chronic illness: visual impairments

Comments: Provides guide dogs to blind persons regardless of race, creed, age, or sex.

PILOT PARENTS
3610 Dodge St., Ste. 101
Omaha, NE 68131
402-346-5220
402-346-5253

Type of organization: nonprofit
Public served: individuals/families, general public, media, nonmedical professionals
Offers: information, reference material, publication(s), support group(s), counseling, seminars/workshops
Disability/chronic illness: mental disabilities

Comments: Group trains parents to help other parents of handicapped children in times of special need. Although local in scope, the group acts as a model for similar groups currently being organized.

PRIDE FOUNDATION (Promote Real Independence for the Disabled and Elderly)
391 Long Hill Rd.
Box 1293
Groton, CT 06340
203-445-1448

Type of organization: nonprofit
Public served: individuals/families, general public, media, non-medical professionals
Offers: information, reference material, publication(s), consultations/guidance, seminars/workshops, products
Disability/chronic illness: physical disabilities

Comments: Provides rehabilitation assistance in the areas of home management, independent dressing, and personal grooming. Designs and develops special garments that will help the handicapped feel more comfortable and dress independently; designs assistive devices for use in the home. Works with any group involved with these individuals.

PULMONARY AND CYSTIC FIBROSIS CENTER
St. Christopher's Hospital
for Children
2600 North Lawrence St.
Philadelphia, PA 19133
215-427-5183

Type of organization: medical facility, research facility
Public served: individuals/families, general public, media, medical personnel
Offers: information, reference material, publication(s), consultations/guidance, seminars/workshops, research material
Disability/chronic illness: cystic fibrosis

R

RECLAMATION, INC.
2502 Waterford
San Antonio, TX 78217
210-824-8618

Type of organization: nonprofit
Public served: individuals/families, general public, media
Offers: information, reference material, publication(s), support group(s), consultations/guidance, civil rights assistance/advocacy
Disability/chronic illness: mental illness

Comments: Members include former mental health patients and interested others. Seeks to eliminate the stigma of mental illness and reclaim members' "human dignity." Serves as a unified voice for mental health patients in consumer, social, and political affairs. Helps members to live outside a hospital setting by providing assistance in the areas of resocialization, employment, and housing. Monitors media coverage; encourages positive presentations of mental health patients and increased coverage of mental health community service projects and events. Acts as a political force in the field. Maintains library of books written by mental health patients. Bestows awards and maintains speakers bureau.

RECORDING FOR THE BLIND
20 Rozel Rd.
Princeton, NJ 08540
1–800–221–4792
609–452–0606
FAX: 609–987–8116

Type of organization: nonprofit
Public served: individuals/families
Offers: information, publication(s)
Disability/chronic illness: visual impairments

Comments: Provides library services, computerized books, books on audiotape, and other educational materials free of charge to those who cannot read standard print. Materials recorded at 31 recording studios by more than 4,800 volunteers. Seeks to supplement, not duplicate materials available through Library of Congress. Has 79,000-volume library.

RECOVERY, THE ASSOCIATION OF NERVOUS AND FORMER MENTAL PATIENTS
802 North Dearborn St.
Chicago, IL 60610
312–337–5661

Type of organization: nonprofit
Public served: individuals/families
Offers: information, publication(s), support group(s)
Disability/chronic illness: mental illness

REGISTRY OF INTERPRETERS FOR THE DEAF
8719 Colesville Rd., #310
Silver Spring, MD 20910
301–608–0050
FAX: 301–608–0508

Type of organization: professional
Public served: individuals/families
Offers: supportive services

Disability/chronic illness: hearing impairments

Comments: Produces list of professional interpreters for the deaf.

REHABILITATION ENGINEERING PROGRAM
345 East Superior St., Rm. 1441
Chicago, IL 60611
312–649–8560

Type of organization: research facility
Public served: individuals/families
Offers: products, living aids
Disability/chronic illness: amputations, arthritis, physical disabilities

Comments: Develops prosthetics, orthotics, and total joint replacements.

REHABILITATION INTERNATIONAL
25 East 21st St.
New York, NY 10010
212–420–1500

Type of organization: nonprofit
Public served: intermediate parties
Offers: information, publication(s), civil rights assistance/advocacy
Disability/chronic illness: all

RESEARCH TO PREVENT BLINDNESS
598 Madison Ave.
New York, NY 10022
1–800–621–0026 (in U.S., except NY)
212–752–4333

Type of organization: nonprofit
Public served: individuals/families, general public, medical personnel, nonmedical professionals, researchers
Offers: information, education, reference material, research material
Disability/chronic illness: visual impairments

Comments: National voluntary health organization that seeks to stimulate basic and applied research into the causes, prevention, and treatment of blinding eye diseases.

RESNA (REHABILITATION ENGINEERING SOCIETY OF NORTH AMERICA)
1101 Connecticut Ave. NW, Ste. 700
Washington, DC 20036
202–857–1199
FAX: 202–223–4579

Type of organization: nonprofit
Public served: individuals/families, general public, media, medical personnel, nonmedical professionals, researchers, intermediate parties
Offers: information, reference material, publication(s), research material, products, living aids
Disability/chronic illness: physical disabilities

Comments: Interdisciplinary association of rehabilitation professionals, providers, and consumers, for the advancement of rehabilitation and assistive technologies. Seeks to improve the quality of life through the application of science and technology, and to influence policy relating to the delivery of technology to disabled persons.

RESOURCES FOR ARTISTS WITH DISABILITIES, INC.
77 Seventh Ave., Ste. PHG
New York, NY 10011–6645
212–691–5490
FAX: 212–255–0615

Type of organization: nonprofit
Public served: individuals/families

Offers: information, publication(s)
Disability/chronic illness: all

Comments: Works to assist disabled artists in the visual arts to exhibit their work. Newsletter includes information on exhibitions and opportunities to exhibit as well as information on grants and art services. At present they have slides on more than 100 artists and their work, which they use to promote their exhibits and to show to other curators. Holds two to four exhibits a year.

ROSE F. KENNEDY CENTER FOR RESEARCH IN MENTAL RETARDATION AND HUMAN DEVELOPMENT
1410 Pelham Pky. South
Bronx, NY 10461
212–430–2413

Type of organization: research facility
Public served: individuals/families, general public, medical personnel
Offers: information, medical referrals, consultations/guidance, seminars/workshops, research material

Disability/chronic illness: mental retardation

RP FOUNDATION FIGHTING BLINDNESS

1401 Mt. Royal Ave., 4th Fl.
Baltimore, MD 21217–4245
1–800–638–5555
410–225–9400*
FAX: 410–225–3936

Type of organization: nonprofit
Public served: individuals/families, general public, medical personnel, researchers
Offers: information, reference material, publication(s), support group(s), medical referrals, nonmedical referrals, research material
Disability/chronic illness: visual impairments

Comments: *410–225–9409 (TDD). Raises funds for research into retinal degenerative diseases, coordinates a retina-donor and registry program as well as self-help networks for those with Usher syndrome and Bardet-Biedl syndrome.

S

SAFE (SELF-ABUSE FINALLY ENDS)

c/o Karen Conterio
P.O. Box 267810
Chicago, IL 60626
1–800–DONTCUT
312–722–3113

Type of organization: nonprofit
Public served: individuals/families
Offers: support group(s)
Disability/chronic illness: mental illness

Comments: Self-help group assisting self-injurious individuals in the treatment of their addictive behavior patterns. Maintains speakers bureau; compiles statistics.

SCHIZOPHRENICS ANONYMOUS

1209 California Rd.
Eastchester, NY 10709
914–337–2252

Type of organization: nonprofit
Public served: individuals/families
Offers: support group(s)

Disability/chronic illness: schizophrenia, mental illness

Comments: A self-help organization sponsored by American Schizophrenia Association. Groups are comprised of diagnosed schizophrenics who meet to share experiences, strengths, and hopes in an effort to help each other cope with common problems and recover from the disease. Rehabilitation program follows the Twelve-Step Program from Alcoholics Anonymous World Services.

SCLERODERMA FOUNDATION, INC.
1377 K St. NW, Ste. 700
Washington, DC 20005
703-938-2191

Type of organization: nonprofit
Public served: individuals/families, general public, media, medical personnel, researchers
Offers: information, education, publication(s), support group(s), research material
Disability/chronic illness: scleroderma

SCLERODERMA INTERNATIONAL FOUNDATION
704 Gardner Center Rd.
New Castle, PA 16101
412-652-3109

Type of organization: nonprofit
Public served: individuals/families, researchers
Offers: information, support group(s), research material
Disability/chronic illness: scleroderma

SCOLIOSIS ASSOCIATION
1 Penn Plaza
New York, NY 10119
212-845-1760

Type of organization: nonprofit
Public served: individuals/families, general public, media
Offers: information, education, support group(s)
Disability/chronic illness: scoliosis, spinal deviations

SCRIPPS CLINIC AND RESEARCH FOUNDATION
10666 North Torrey Pines Rd.
La Jolla, CA 92037
619-455-9100

Type of organization: medical facility, research facility
Public served: individuals/families, general public, media, medical personnel, nonmedical professionals
Offers: information, education, reference material, medical services, consultations/guidance, research material

97

Disability/chronic illness: chronic pain

Comments: Has a trauma center in addition to standard medical facilities. Well known for progressive approach to treatment.

SEEING EYE, THE
Box 375
Morristown, NJ 07960
201-539-4425

Type of organization: nonprofit
Public served: individuals/families, general public, media, medical personnel, nonmedical professionals
Offers: information, education, publication(s), counseling, living aids, independent living assistance
Disability/chronic illness: visual impairments

Comments: Provides guide dogs.

SHEALY PAIN AND HEALTH REHABILITATION INSTITUTE
3525 South National
Springfield, MO 65807
417-882-0850

Type of organization: nonprofit
Public served: individuals/families, general public, media
Offers: information, education, reference material, publica-

tion(s), medical services, consultations/guidance, seminars/workshops
Disability/chronic illness: chronic pain

SHRINERS BURNS INSTITUTE
202 Goodman St.
Cincinnati, OH 45219
1-800-237-5055
513-751-3900

Type of organization: medical facility
Public served: individuals/families, general public, media, medical personnel, researchers
Offers: information, support group(s), counseling, medical services, research material, rehabilitative services
Disability/chronic illness: severe burns

Comments: Children only.

SIBLING INFORMATION NETWORK
c/o A. J. Pappanikou Center
1776 Ellington Rd.
South Windsor, CT 06074
203-648-1205
FAX: 203-644-2031

Type of organization: nonprofit
Public served: individuals/families, general public, media, nonmedical professionals

Offers: information, publica-
tion(s), support group(s),
counseling
Disability/chronic illness: developmental disabilities

Comments: For teachers, social
workers, health care professionals, researchers, and families who
have an interest in the welfare of
siblings of children with disabilities and issues related to families
of individuals with disabilities.
Acts as clearinghouse for information and services regarding the siblings of persons with handicaps.

SIBLINGS OF
DISABLED CHILDREN
535 Race St., Ste. 120
San Jose, CA 95126
408–288–5010
FAX: 408–288–7943

Type of organization: nonprofit
Public served: individuals/families
Offers: information, support
group(s), counseling
Disability/chronic illness: all

Comments: A division of Parents
Helping Parents; organization was
established to address the needs of
siblings of chronically ill or disabled children and to provide them
with a support system. Works to
enable them to express their emotions about the ill or disabled

sibling and the situation in a therapeutic environment.

SIBLINGS FOR
SIGNIFICANT CHANGE
105 East 22nd St., 7th Fl.
New York, NY 10010
212–420–0776
FAX: 212–420–0433

Type of organization: nonprofit
Public served: individuals/families,
medical personnel, nonmedical
professionals
Offers: information, support
group(s), counseling
Disability/chronic illness: all

Comments: Directed to the siblings
of disabled children as well as parents, educators, social workers,
medical professionals, and researchers. Provides peer support,
legal assistance, and psychological counseling to siblings of the
handicapped. Coordinates social
activities for families with handicapped members and works on
projects to increase public awareness of these families' difficulties.

SICKLE CELL DISEASE
ASSOCIATION OF AMERICA
3345 Wilshire Blvd.
Los Angeles, CA 90010
1–800–421–8453
213–736–5455
FAX: 213–736–5211

Type of organization: nonprofit
Public served: individuals/families, general public, media
Offers: information, publication(s), support group(s), medical referrals, nonmedical referrals, seminars/workshops, financial assistance, research material
Disability/chronic illness: sickle cell anemia

SISTER KENNY INSTITUTE
800 East 28th St.
(at Chicago Ave.)
Minneapolis, MN 55407
612–874–4463

Type of organization: medical facility
Public served: individuals/families, general public, media, medical personnel
Offers: information, diagnostic services, publication(s), medical services, consultations/guidance, research material, rehabilitative services, vocational services
Disability/chronic illness: neurological diseases, musculoskeletal disorders

SKI FOR LIGHT
1445 West Lake St.
Minneapolis, MN 55408
612–827–3232

Type of organization: nonprofit
Public served: individuals/families, general public
Offers: information, reference material, publication(s), consultations/guidance, seminars/workshops, recreational opportunities
Disability/chronic illness: visual impairments, physical disabilities

Comments: Encourages cross-country skiing and other sports activities for visually impaired and physically disabled. Works to help organize new groups.

SOCIETY FOR THE ADVANCEMENT OF TRAVEL FOR THE HANDICAPPED
347 5th Ave., Ste. 610
New York, NY 10016
212–447–7284
FAX: 212–725–8253

Type of organization: nonprofit
Public served: individuals/families, general public, media, nonmedical professionals
Offers: information, reference material, publication(s), seminars/workshops, travel assistance
Disability/chronic illness: all

Comments: Individuals and corporations interested in creating a forum for the exchange of ideas, information, and resources to encourage and ease travel for handicapped persons. Goals: to increase awareness of the need and ability of handicapped persons to travel, to have them welcomed, and to act as a resource center for related information.

SPECIAL OLYMPICS, INC.
1350 New York Ave. NW, #500
Washington, DC 20005
202–628–3630
FAX: 202–737–1937

Type of organization: nonprofit
Public served: individuals/families, general public, media
Offers: information, recreational opportunities
Disability/chronic illness: mental retardation

Comments: Local chapters. Works to promote physical fitness, sports training, and athletic competition for the mentally retarded from age 8 through adulthood. Competitions held from local to international levels in track and field, swimming, gymnastics, bowling, ice skating, basketball and others. Provides information on programs and has speakers bureau.

SPECIAL RECREATION, INC.
362 Koser Ave.
Iowa City, IA 52246–3038
319–337–7578
FAX: 319–338–3320

Type of organization: nonprofit
Public served: individuals/families, nonmedical professionals
Offers: information, support group(s), consultations/guidance, recreational opportunities, civil rights assistance/advocacy, research material
Disability/chronic illness: all

Comments: Members include disabled consumers, parents of the disabled, rehabilitation professionals, and volunteers. Supports, encourages, and promotes self-determination, equal opportunity, consumerism, and normalization in recreation and leisure for disabled individuals. Conducts research and demonstrations, prepares and disseminates information, cooperates with and assists voluntary associations and public agencies in initiating, expanding, and improving special recreation programs and services, and provides personnel training. Sponsors the International Center on Special Recreation that works to: collect and desseminate international information on special recreation services for disabled persons, special recreation programs and personnel training; conduct, provide, and support international exchange of technical, professional, and general information on social recreation for the disabled; cooperate with both governmental and voluntary organizations on national and international levels. Maintains Pioneers in Special Recreation Hall of Fame and biographical archives. Bestows annual Special Recreation Awards. Offers career guidance and placement service, maintains 4,000-volume library and speakers bureau, and compiles statistics.

SPINAL CORD SOCIETY

2410 Lakeview Dr.
Fergus Falls, MN 56537
1–800–328–8253
1–800–862–0179 (in MN)

Type of organization: nonprofit
Public served: individuals/families, general public, media, researchers
Offers: information, medical referrals, civil rights assistance/advocacy, research material
Disability/chronic illness: spinal cord injury, central nervous system injury and disease

Comments: Call 1–800–526–3456 for the hotline. For spinal cord injury prevention information, call 1–800–342–0330. Works to promote research and increase public awareness concerning the potential for a cure of paralysis due to spinal cord injury. Maintains data bank of chronic spinal cord injury case histories as well as a medical center in Minneapolis that uses state-of-the-art treatments for paralysis victims.

STATE VOCATIONAL REHABILITATION AGENCIES*

Type of organization: government
Public served: individuals/families
Offers: information, counseling, financial assistance, rehabilitative services, vocational services
Disability/chronic illness: all

Comments: *See local government listings for your state to find the nearest office.

SUPPORT DOGS FOR THE HANDICAPPED
301 Sovereign Ct., Ste. 113
St. Louis, MO 63011
314-394-6163

Type of organization: nonprofit
Public served: individuals/families
Offers: information, education, living aids
Disability/chronic illness: all

Comments: For veterinarians, dog trainers, and people with disabilities, medical- and animal-oriented organizations, and interested individuals. Helps people with functional limitations achieve greater independence and improve the quality of their lives by providing them with professionally trained support and TOUCH dogs.

T

TASH: ASSOCIATION FOR PERSONS WITH SEVERE HANDICAPS
11201 Greenwood Ave. North
Seattle, WA 98133
206-361-8870
FAX: 206-361-9208

Type of organization: nonprofit
Public served: individuals/families,
general public, media, non-medical professionals
Offers: information, reference material, publication(s), consultations/guidance, civil rights assistance/advocacy
Disability/chronic illness: all

Comments: Members include teachers, therapists, parents, administrators, university faculty, lawyers, and advocates involved in all areas of service to people with severe disabilities. Seeks to ensure an autonomous, dignified lifestyle, and quality education for those with severe disabilities.

TOURETTE SYNDROME ASSOCIATION
41-02 Bell Blvd.
Bayside, NY 11361
1-800-237-0717
212-224-2999

Type of organization: nonprofit
Public served: individuals/families, general public, media, medical personnel, researchers
Offers: information, medical referrals, civil rights assistance/advocacy, research material
Disability/chronic illness: Tourette syndrome

TRAVEL INDUSTRY DISABLED EXCHANGE (TIDE)
5435 Donna Ave.
Tarzana, CA 91356
818–343–6339

Type of organization: nonprofit
Public served: individuals/families, general public, media, non-medical professionals
Offers: information, publication(s), seminars/workshops, travel assistance
Disability/chronic illness: all

Comments: Travel industry personnel and disabled individuals united to enhance travel opportunities for the disabled. Conducts seminars, surveys travel facilities for the disabled.

U

U.S. ARCHITECTURAL AND TRANSPORTATION BARRIERS COMPLIANCE BOARD
1331 F St. NW, Ste. 1000
Washington, DC 20004
1–800–USA–ABLE
  (voice or TDD)
202–272–5434 (voice)*

Type of organization: government
Public served: individuals/families
Offers: information
Disability/chronic illness: all

Comments: *202–272–5449 (TDD). Disseminates technical information and assistance on creating a barrier-free environment to federal, state, and local government agencies and to private organizations and individuals.

UNITED CEREBRAL PALSY ASSOCIATIONS, INC.
1522 K St. NW, Ste. 1112
Washington, DC 20005–1202
1–800–872–5827
202–842–1266
FAX: 202–842–3519

Type of organization: nonprofit
Public served: individuals/families, general public, media
Offers: information, publication(s), support group(s), medical referrals, seminars/workshops
Disability/chronic illness: cerebral palsy

Comments: Has local chapters nationwide that provide programs and services.

UNITED SCLERODERMA FOUNDATION, INC.
P.O. Box 350
Watsonville, CA 95077–0350
1–800–722–HOPE
408–728–2202

Type of organization: nonprofit
Public served: individuals/families,
 general public, media
Offers: information, publica-
 tion(s), support group(s),
 medical referrals, seminars/
 workshops, research material
Disability/chronic illness: scleroderma, arthritis

Comments: Has local chapters nationwide.

UNITED STATES ASSOCIATION FOR BLIND ATHLETES

33 North Institute St.
Colorado Springs, CO 80903
719–630–0422
FAX: 719–578–4654

Type of organization: nonprofit
Public served: individuals/families,
 general public
Offers: information, publica-
 tion(s), consultations/guid-
 ance, seminars/workshops,
 recreational opportunities
Disability/chronic illness: visual
 impairments

Comments: Trains, coaches and
prepares blind athletes for national
and international sports competition, winter and summer. Sports
include alpine skiing, goalball,
gymnastics, judo, nordic skiing,
powerlifting, speed skating, swim-

ming, tandem cycling, track and
field, and wrestling.

UNITED STATES DEAF SKIERS ASSOCIATION

c/o Sandra McGee
130 Rosewood Pl.
Bridgeport, CT 06610
517–646–6811 (TDD)

Type of organization: nonprofit
Public served: individuals/families
Offers: information, recreational
 opportunities
Disability/chronic illness: hearing
 impairments

Comments: Promotes recreational
and competitive skiing for deaf
persons. Provides deaf skiers with
benefits, activities, and opportunities that will increase their enjoy-
ment of the sport. Sponsors
regional and national races, assists
in the selection, organization, and
training of the U.S. Deaf Ski
Team for international competition.

UNITED STATES ORGANIZATION FOR DISABLED ATHLETES

c/o John Hurley
143 California Ave.
Uniondale, NY 11553–1131
516–485–3701
FAX: 516–485–3707

Type of organization: nonprofit
Public served: individuals/families, general public, media
Offers: information, recreational opportunities
Disability/chronic illness: all

Comments: Coordinates services for the disabled, their coaches, and those interested in disabled athletes. Seeks to enhance the self-esteem, proficiency, and daily lives of physically disabled children, youth, and adults. Conducts the Disabled Youth Awareness Program and is involved in the Physically Disabled Winter Sports Festival, and the Paralympics, which coincide with the Olympic Games.

UNITED WAY OF AMERICA
701 North Fairfax St.
Alexandria, VA 22314–2088
703–836–7100
FAX: 703–683–7840

Type of organization: nonprofit
Public served: individuals/families, intermediate parties
Offers: information, medical referrals, nonmedical referrals
Disability/chronic illness: all

Comments: Has local chapters. Disburses funds to various service providers in the community to assist in meeting needs of a wide variety of clients, from handicapped and disabled to abused women. Check your local chapter for information and referral to services, some of which may be unique to your community.

U.S. DEPARTMENT OF AGRICULTURE
Farmers Home Administration, Home Loans
Washington, DC 20250
202–720–7967
FAX: 202–720–7967

Type of organization: government
Public served: individuals/families
Offers: information, financial assistance, housing
Disability/chronic illness: all

Comments: Section 502 Rural Housing Loans provide for those with very low to moderate incomes. Offers direct loans, guaranteed/insured loans. Check local telephone directory for area office.

U.S. DEPARTMENT OF AGRICULTURE
Farmers Home Administration, Housing Repair Loans and Grants
Single-Family Housing Processing Division
Washington, DC 20250
202–720–1474
FAX: 202–720–1474

Type of organization: government
Public served: individuals/families
Offers: financial assistance,
   housing
Disability/chronic illness: all

Comments: Direct loans, project grants available for homeowners in rural areas to repair or improve their dwellings. Check local directory for area office.

U.S. DEPARTMENT OF AGRICULTURE

Farmers Home Administration,
   Housing Site Loans
Single-Family Housing
   Processing Division
Washington, DC 20250
202–720–1474
FAX: 202–720–1474

Type of organization: government
Public served: individuals/families
Offers: financial assistance,
   housing
Disability/chronic illness: all

Comments: Sections 523 and 524 Site Loans. Direct loans go to private or public nonprofit organizations that will provide the developed sites to qualified borrowers. Check local directory for area office.

U.S. DEPARTMENT OF AGRICULTURE

Farmers Home Administration,
   Rental Assistance
Multi-family Housing Services
   and Property Management
   Division
Washington, DC 20250
202–720–1599
FAX: 202–720–1599

Type of organization: government
Public served: individuals/families
Offers: information, financial
   assistance, housing
Disability/chronic illness: all

Comments: Direct payments available to reduce rent for very low- and low-income families and handicapped or senior citizens in eligible rental housing. Check local directory for area office.

U.S. DEPARTMENT OF AGRICULTURE

Farmers Home Administration,
   Rural Housing Preservation
   Grants
Multiple Family Housing
   Processing Division
Washington, DC 20250
202–720–1606
FAX: 202–720–1606

Type of organization: government
Public served: individuals/families, intermediate parties
Offers: information, financial assistance, housing
Disability/chronic illness: all

Comments: Project grants to intermediate parties to give very-low- and low-income rural homeowners assistance to provide needed repairs to their homes. Check local directory for area offices.

U.S. DEPARTMENT OF AGRICULTURE
Farmers Home Administration,
   Rural Rental Housing Loans
Director, Multi-Family Housing
   Processing Division
Washington, DC 20250
202–382–1604
FAX: 202–382–1604

Type of organization: government
Public served: individuals/families, general public
Offers: financial assistance, housing
Disability/chronic illness: all

Comments: Direct loans go to qualified applicants for multi-family units for very low-, low- or moderate-income families, senior citizens, or the handicapped. Check local directory for area office.

U.S. DEPARTMENT OF AGRICULTURE
Farmers Home Administration,
   Self-Help Technical Assistance
Single-Family Housing
   Processing Division
Washington, DC 20250
202–720–1474
FAX: 202–720–1474

Type of organization: government
Public served: individuals/families
Offers: information, financial assistance, housing
Disability/chronic illness: all

Comments: Project grants for technical and supervisory assistance to aid needy very low- and low-income individuals in carrying out mutual self-help projects in rural areas. Check local directory for area office.

U.S. DEPARTMENT OF AGRICULTURE
Food and Nutrition Service
Director, Child Nutrition
   Division
Alexandria, VA 22302
703–305–2590
FAX: 703–305–2590

Type of organization: government
Public served: individuals/families, intermediate parties
Offers: food

Disability/chronic illness: mental or physical handicaps

Comments: Child and Adult Care Food Program. Local organizations or agencies who meet eligibility criteria receive funds for meals for qualified individuals. (An example is an institution providing day-care services for the handicapped.)

U.S. DEPARTMENT OF AGRICULTURE

Food and Nutrition Service,
Food Donation Program
Food Distribution Division
Alexandria, VA 22302
703–305–2680
FAX: 703–305–2680

Type of organization: government
Public served: individuals/families, intermediate parties
Offers: food
Disability/chronic illness: all

Comments: Food distributed through qualified organizations or agencies and served to needy individuals and families. Restrictions apply. Check local directory for regional office of Food and Nutrition Service.

U.S. DEPARTMENT OF AGRICULTURE

Food and Nutrition Service
Food Stamp Program
Alexandria, VA 22302
703–305–2026

Type of organization: government
Public served: individuals/families, intermediate parties
Offers: financial assistance, food
Disability/chronic illness: all

Comments: Households apply through local Department of Human Services office and are determined to be in need of food assistance. Qualifying factors may include unemployment, part-time employment, limited pension or low wages. Check local directory for office nearest you.

U.S. DEPARTMENT OF AGRICULTURE

Food and Nutrition Service
Park Office Center, Rm. 502
3101 Park Center Dr.
Alexandria, VA 22302
703–305–2680

Type of organization: government
Public served: individuals/families, intermediate parties

Offers: food
Disability/chronic illness: all

Comments: Food commodities are distributed through the states and then to local agencies providing food to needy individuals, whether they are unemployed, welfare recipients, or have low incomes. Check with local Department of Human Services, United Way Agency, Office of Information and Referral, Senior Citizens Center, or county courthouse.

U.S. DEPARTMENT OF AGRICULTURE
Food and Nutrition Service
Supplemental Food Programs
   Division
Alexandria, VA 22302
703–305–2746
FAX: 703–305–2746

Type of organization: government
Public served: individuals/families,
   intermediate parties
Offers: food
Disability/chronic illness: all

Comments: Supplemental nutritious foods are provided to pregnant and postpartum women, infants, and children up to 5 years of age who are determined to be at nutritional risk. Intermediary agencies participate in the Women, Infants, and Children (WIC) Program. Check with the local Department of Human Services or the regional Food and Nutrition Service office.

U.S. DEPARTMENT OF EDUCATION
Postsecondary Education
Regional Office Bldg. 3
7th and D Sts. SW
Washington, DC 20202–5251
202–708–4653

Type of organization: government
Public served: individuals/families,
   intermediate parties
Offers: education, financial
   assistance
Disability/chronic illness: all

Comments: Legal Training for the Disadvantaged program assists minority, low-income and educationally disadvantaged college graduates to undertake training in the legal profession. Though not specifically stated, handicapped individuals may qualify under low-income guidelines or as educationally disadvantaged. Contact the Washington office.

U.S. DEPARTMENT OF EDUCATION
Postsecondary Education
Washington, DC 20202–5251
202–708–7861

110

Type of organization: government
Public served: individuals/families,
   intermediate parties
Offers: education
Disability/chronic illness: all

Comments: Veterans Education
Outreach Program's objective is
to assist colleges and universities
in serving the special needs of veterans, especially the physically
disabled or educationally disadvantaged veterans. This assistance
may include outreach, recruit-
ment, counseling, tutoring, or
special education. Call the veterans services office at your school.

U.S. DEPARTMENT OF EDUCATION

Postsecondary Education
400 Maryland Ave. SW
Washington, DC 20202–5446
202–708–4690

Type of organization: government
Public served: individuals/families
Offers: education, financial
   assistance
Disability/chronic illness: all or
   none

Comments: Offers Federal Supplemental Educational Opportunity
Grants to provide grant assistance
for eligible undergraduate postsecondary students with demon-

strated financial need. Open to
anyone, not just handicapped. For
specific eligibility, contact the educational institution financial aid
office.

U.S. DEPARTMENT OF EDUCATION

Postsecondary Education
400 Maryland Ave. SW
Washington, DC 20202
202–708–4607

Type of organization: government
Public served: individuals/families,
   intermediate parties
Offers: education, financial
   assistance
Disability/chronic illness: all

Comments: The Pell Grant program provides eligible undergraduate postsecondary students who
have demonstrated financial need
with grant assistance to help meet
educational expenses. Open to
any individual who meets certain
criteria. Contact the financial aid
office of your school.

U.S. DEPARTMENT OF EDUCATION

Postsecondary Education
400 Maryland Ave. SW
Washington, DC 20202
202–708–4690

Type of organization: government
Public served: individuals/families,
    intermediate parties
Offers: education, financial
    assistance
Disability/chronic illness: all

Comments: The federal work-study program works to provide part-time employment to eligible postsecondary students to help meet educational expenses. Also encourages students receiving program assistance to participate in community service activities. Contact the financial aid office at your educational institution.

U.S. DEPARTMENT OF EDUCATION

Postsecondary Education
400 Maryland Ave. SW
Washington, DC 20202
202–708–4804

Type of organization: government
Public served: individuals/families,
    intermediate parties
Offers: supportive services
Disability/chronic illness: all

Comments: Student Support Services Project Grants work to provide supportive services to disadvantaged college students to enhance their potential for successfully completing postsecondary education. This can include

tutoring, mentoring, or assisting disabled students. Contact the disabled students office at your educational institution.

U.S. DEPARTMENT OF EDUCATION

Postsecondary Education
400 Maryland Ave. SW
Washington, DC 20202
202–708–8242

Type of organization: government
Public served: individuals/families,
    intermediate parties
Offers: education, financial
    assistance
Disability/chronic illness: all

Comments: Perkins Loan Program works to provide low-interest loans for undergraduate, graduate, or professional students who have shown financial need and are enrolled in or accepted for enrollment as regular students in an eligible program at a postsecondary educational institution. Contact the financial aid office of your school.

U.S. DEPARTMENT OF EDUCATION

Postsecondary Education
Policy Development, Policy,
    Training and Analysis Service
Washington, DC 20202
202–708–8242

Type of organization: government
Public served: individuals/families, intermediate parties
Offers: education, financial assistance
Disability/chronic illness: all

Comments: Guaranteed Student Loans are available to anyone who is enrolled in a degree or certificate program on at least a half-time basis as an undergraduate, graduate, or professional student at a participating postsecondary school. Contact the financial aid office of the school or the national headquarters for a listing of participating institutions.

U.S. DEPARTMENT OF EDUCATION

Special Education and
  Rehabilitative Services
330 C St. SW
Washington, DC 20202-2575
202-205-8352
202-205-8352 (TDD)

Type of organization: government
Public served: individuals/families, intermediate parties
Offers: independent living assistance
Disability/chronic illness: severe physical or mental impairments, which keep the individual from functioning independently in the family or in the community or which substantially limit employment

Comments: Centers for Independent Living provides a network of centers for independent living and includes such services as information and referral, training in independent living skills, peer counseling, and individual and systems advocacy. Contact state rehabilitative office.

U.S. DEPARTMENT OF EDUCATION

Special Education and
  Rehabilitative Services
400 Maryland Ave. SW
Washington, DC 20202
202-205-5809

Type of organization: government
Public served: individuals/families, intermediate parties
Offers: education
Disability/chronic illness: all (in infants and youth)

Comments: Regional resource and federal centers that provide advice and technical services for improving education of children with disabilities. Such centers are usually established at higher education institutions, state education agencies, public agencies, and private nonprofit organizations.

113

U.S. DEPARTMENT OF EDUCATION

Special Education and
   Rehabilitative Services
400 Maryland Ave. SW
Washington, DC 20202
202-205-5809

Type of organization: government
Public served: individuals/families,
   intermediate parties
Offers: education
Disability/chronic illness: visual and
   hearing impairments

Comments: Has Services for Children with Deaf-Blindness programs. Seeks to provide state education agencies with technical assistance in order to improve services to deaf-blind children and youth. There is no direct aid to individuals/families but parents should check with local education districts for more information on any services that have come under the program.

U.S. DEPARTMENT OF EDUCATION

Special Education and
   Rehabilitative Services
400 Maryland Ave. SW
Washington, DC 20202
202-205-5809

Type of organization: government
Public served: individuals/families,
   general public, media, medical personnel, nonmedical professionals, intermediate parties
Offers: information, education
Disability/chronic illness: all

Comments: Clearinghouses for individuals with disabilities. Disseminates information regarding education programs and services for disabled children. Provides technical assistance to professionals and others interested in pursuing a career in special education as well as information on postsecondary education for those with disabilities. Contact the Washington office.

U.S. DEPARTMENT OF EDUCATION

Special Education and
   Rehabilitative Services
400 Maryland Ave. SW
Washington, DC 20202
202-205-8163

Type of organization: government
Public served: individuals/families,
   intermediate parties
Offers: education
Disability/chronic illness: all

Comments: Postsecondary Education Programs for Persons with Disabilities seeks to develop, operate, and disseminate specially designed vocational, technical, postsecondary, or adult education model programs for deaf or other disabled persons. Contact the Washington office to determine if there are any programs established at an educational institution near you.

U.S. DEPARTMENT OF EDUCATION
Special Education and
    Rehabilitative Services
400 Maryland Ave. SW
Washington, DC 20202
202–205–8825

Type of organization: government
Public served: individuals/families
Offers: education
Disability/chronic illness: mental retardation; hearing, speech or language impairments; visual handicaps, serious emotional disturbance; orthopedic handicaps; other impairments

Comments: Chapter 1, ESEA Handicapped provides programs that supplement services to children who are disabled and enrolled in state-operated or state-supported schools. Also programs for children who are disabled and enrolled in local education agencies who have transferred from a state school or program. Contact state coordinator for the program at the state department of education.

U.S. DEPARTMENT OF EDUCATION
Special Education and
    Rehabilitative Services
400 Maryland Ave. SW
Washington, DC 20202
202–205–8825

Type of organization: government
Public served: individuals/families, intermediate parties
Offers: education
Disability/chronic illness: mental, physical, emotional or learning disabilities

Comments: Special education, state grants are available to assist states in providing free, appropriate public education to all children with disabilities in each state as well as those in the District of Columbia, Puerto Rico, American Samoa, Mariana Islands, Guam, Virgin Islands, Marshall Islands, and Palau. Contact the local schools.

U.S. DEPARTMENT OF EDUCATION

Special Education and
  Rehabilitative Services
400 Maryland Ave. SW
Washington, DC 20202
202–205–9084

Type of organization: government
Public served: individuals/families,
  intermediate parties
Offers: information, diagnostic
  services, publication(s),
  medical referrals, non-
  medical referrals, medical
  services
Disability/chronic illness: all

Comments: Operates Grants for Infants and Toddlers with Disabilities for Early Intervention program. States will develop a statewide comprehensive, coordinated multidisciplinary interagency system to provide early intervention services for all children with disabilities, ages birth to 2 years, and their families. Check with your doctor, county health department MH/MR agency, or social workers at hospitals or state school.

U.S. DEPARTMENT OF EDUCATION

Special Education and
  Rehabilitative Services
400 Maryland Ave. SW
Washington, DC 20202
202–205–9084

Type of organization: government
Public served: individuals/families,
  intermediate parties
Offers: education
Disability/chronic illness: all

Comments: Grants to states to assist them in providing a free appropriate public education to preschool disabled children ages 3–5. Contact your local school district.

U.S. DEPARTMENT OF EDUCATION

Special Education and
  Rehabilitative Services
Washington, DC 20202
202–205–9406

Type of organization: government
Public served: individuals/families,
  intermediate parties
Offers: rehabilitative services,
  vocational services
Disability/chronic illness: all

Comments: Vocational Rehabilitation Services Program assists each state in operating comprehensive vocational rehabilitation programs that are accountable to the federal government. Designed to assess, plan, develop, and provide such services for disabled persons, consistent with their strengths, resources, priorities, concerns, abilities, and capabilities. Helps them to prepare for and engage in competitive employment. Contact the state's rehabilitative services office.

U.S. DEPARTMENT OF EDUCATION

Special Education and
  Rehabilitative Services
Switzer Bldg., Rm. 4615
400 Maryland Ave. SW
Washington, DC 20202
202–205–5809

Type of organization: government
Public served: individuals/families,
  intermediate parties
Offers: education
Disability/chronic illness: severe disabilities (in infants and youth)

Comments: Severely Disabled program seeks to address the special education, related services, and early intervention needs of children and youth with severe disabilities. Grants are made to public and private, profit and nonprofit, organizations and institutions. Contact the Washington office to determine if any programs are offered in your area.

U.S. DEPARTMENT OF EDUCATION

Special Education and
  Rehabilitative Services
Division of Educational Services
Washington, DC 20202
202–205–9172
202–205–8170 (TDD)

Type of organization: government
Public served: individuals/families,
  intermediate parties
Offers: education
Disability/chronic illness: all

Comments: Operates Media and Captioning for Individuals with Disabilities program, maintains a free loan service of captioned films for the deaf and instructional media for the educational, cultural, and vocational enrichment of the disabled. Provides for purchase and distribution of media materials and equipment. These are in support of efforts made by any educational institution, regardless of profit status.

U.S. DEPARTMENT OF EDUCATION

Special Education and
  Rehabilitative Services
400 Maryland Ave. SW
Washington, DC 20202
202–205–9796

Type of organization: government
Public served: individuals/families, intermediate parties
Offers: vocational services
Disability/chronic illness: physical, mental, learning, or emotional disabilities

Comments: Projects with Industry program creates and expands job and career opportunities in the competitive labor market and provides appropriate placement resources by engaging private industry in training and placement. Grants go to employers, labor unions, profit-making and nonprofit organizations, institutions, and state vocational rehabilitation agencies. Contact state rehabilitation offices.

U.S. DEPARTMENT OF EDUCATION

Special Education and
   Rehabilitative Services
400 Maryland Ave. SW
Washington, DC 20202–2524
202–205–8241

Type of organization: government
Public served: individuals/families, general public, media, non-medical professionals
Offers: information
Disability/chronic illness: all

Comments: Clearinghouse on Disability Information provides information and data regarding the location, provision, and availability of services and programs for persons with disabilities. Includes information on various disabling conditions. Emphasis is on national information resources, federal assistance to programs for, and federal legislation and regulations affecting, individuals with disabilities.

U.S. DEPARTMENT OF EDUCATION

Special Education and
   Rehabilitative Services
400 Maryland Ave. SW
Washington, DC 20202–2572
202–205–5666

Type of organization: government
Public served: individuals/families, intermediate parties
Offers: living aids
Disability/chronic illness: all

Comments: Technology Assistance Program provides grants to states to assist them in developing and implementing comprehensive, consumer-responsive statewide programs of technology-related assistance for individuals of all ages with disabilities. States may provide assistance to statewide community-based organizations or directly to individuals with disabilities. Contact the state's rehabilitative services office.

U.S. DEPARTMENT OF EDUCATION
Special Education and
    Rehabilitative Services
MES Bldg., Rm. 3038
330 C St. SW
Washington, DC 20202-2741
202-205-8292

Type of organization: government
Public served: individuals/families, intermediate parties
Offers: independent living assistance
Disability/chronic illness: visual impairments

Comments: Independent Living Services for Older Individuals (55 or older) helps those who are blind and whose severe visual impairments make gainful employment extremely difficult to attain, but for whom independent living in their own homes or communities is feasible. Approach state rehabilitative services or commissions for the blind.

U.S. DEPARTMENT OF EDUCATION
Special Education and
    Rehabilitative Services
MES Bldg., Rm. 3326
330 C St. SW
Washington, DC 20202-2575
202-205-9406
202-732-1352 (TDD)

Type of organization: government
Public served: individuals/families, intermediate parties
Offers: civil rights assistance/ advocacy
Disability/chronic illness: all

Comments: Program of Protection and Advocacy of Individual Rights provides grants to states to establish systems for protection and advocacy for the rights of individuals with disabilities. Contact the state's rehabilitative services office or the Washington office.

U.S. DEPARTMENT OF EDUCATION
Special Education and
    Rehabilitative Services
See comments below
Washington, DC 20202-2574
202-205-9406

Type of organization: government
Public served: individuals/families, intermediate parties
Offers: vocational services
Disability/chronic illness: severe disabilities

Comments: State Supported Employment Services Program provides grants to state vocational rehabilitation agencies for time-limited services leading to supported employment for individuals with the most severe disabilities. Grants may be used to provide skilled job trainers, systematic training, job development, etc. Contact local MH/MR agencies, United Way offices, state employment agencies, or state schools.

U.S. DEPARTMENT OF EDUCATION

Special Education and
Rehabilitative Services
See comments below
Washington, DC 20202
202–205–8292

Type of organization: government
Public served: individuals/families, intermediate parties
Offers: independent living assistance
Disability/chronic illness: severe physical or mental impairments

Comments: Independent Living Services, Comprehensive Services, Part B, assists states to promote a philosophy of independent living for those with severe physical or mental impairment. Such services are generally handled by the state rehabilitative office.

U.S. DEPARTMENT OF EDUCATION

Special Education and
Rehabilitative Services
Washington, DC 20202
202–205–9554

Type of organization: government
Public served: individuals/families, nonmedical professionals
Offers: education
Disability/chronic illness: all (in children and youths)

Comments: Has Special Education Personnel Development and Parent Training program. Works to increase the number of special education teachers along with other service providers in special education. Also directed toward providing parent training and information services. Parent organizations contact the Washington office for more information.

U.S. DEPARTMENT OF ENERGY

Conservation and Renewable
  Energy
Forrestal Bldg.
Mail Stop CE-532
Washington, DC 20585
202–586–2204

Type of organization: government
Public served: individuals/families
Offers: financial assistance,
  housing
Disability/chronic illness: all

Comments: Weatherization Assistance for Low-Income Persons provides formula grants to insulate the dwellings of low-income persons, particularly the elderly and handicapped low-income, in order to conserve energy and aid those persons least able to afford higher utility costs. Contact national office for regional offices, phone numbers, and contact persons.

U.S. EQUAL EMPLOYMENT OPPORTUNITY COMMISSION

Office of Communications and
  Legislative Affairs
1801 L St. NW
Washington, DC 20507
1–800–669–3362

Type of organization: government
Public served: individuals/families

Offers: civil rights assistance/
  advocacy, vocational services
Disability/chronic illness: all

Comments: Employment Discrimination—Title I of the Americans with Disabilities Act, Investigations: goal is to provide for enforcement of the federal prohibition against employment discrimination by private employers and state and local governments against qualified individuals with disabilities. Contact the nearest EEOC office.

U.S. EQUAL EMPLOYMENT OPPORTUNITY COMMISSION

Office of Communications and
  Legislative Affairs
1801 L St. NW
Washington, DC 20507
1–800–669–3362

Type of organization: government
Public served: individuals/families,
  general public, media, intermediate parties
Offers: information, publication(s), seminars/workshops, civil rights assistance/
  advocacy
Disability/chronic illness: all

Comments: Implements the Technical Assistance for the Americans with Disabilities Act program, which provides information to help employers, other covered entities, and persons with disabilities learn about their obligations and rights under the employment provisions of the ADA. Contact any EEOC office.

U.S. FEDERAL EMERGENCY MANAGEMENT AGENCY
Emergency Food and Shelter
   Program
701 North Fairfax St., Ste. 310
Alexandria, VA 22314
703–706–9660

Type of organization: government
Public served: individuals/families,
   intermediate parties
Offers: financial assistance,
   housing, food
Disability/chronic illness: all

Comments: There are two programs, one that provides mass shelter and food and one that provides assistance to those in their homes who are experiencing difficulties in keeping their housing and having food. Criteria are established by the local organization overseeing the program. Contact either the local office of FEMA or the local United Way chapter.

U.S. DEPARTMENT OF HEALTH AND HUMAN SERVICES
Administration on Aging
Washington, DC 20201
202–619–0013

Type of organization: government
Public served: individuals/families,
   intermediate parties
Offers: independent living
   assistance
Disability/chronic illness: Alzheimer's disease, neurological
   and organic brain dysfunctions

Comments: In-Home Services provides grants to states for services for frail older individuals. Includes in-home supportive services, personal care, and other state-defined services for older individuals with the above conditions, and their families. Contact regional aging-program directors, Department of Health and Human Services regional office.

U.S. DEPARTMENT OF HEALTH AND HUMAN SERVICES
Administration for Children
   and Families
Children's Bureau
P.O. Box 1182
Washington, DC 20013
202–205–9618

Type of organization: government
Public served: individuals/families,
   intermediate parties
Offers: financial assistance
Disability/chronic illness: all
   (in children)

Comments: Adoption assistance for those adopting children who have special needs; for instance, a physical handicap, which makes it reasonable to conclude that they cannot be adopted without adoption assistance. Contact the regional Health and Human Services office.

U.S. DEPARTMENT OF HEALTH AND HUMAN SERVICES

Administration for Children
   and Families
Aerospace Bldg., 5th Fl.
370 L'Enfant Promenade, SW
Washington, DC 20447
202–401–9275

Type of organization: government
Public served: individuals/families,
   intermediate parties
Offers: financial assistance
Disability/chronic illness: all

Comments: Aid to Families with Dependent Children program is available to needy families with dependent children deprived of parental support or care and families with children needing emergency welfare assistance. Funds go to the states who then disburse them to eligible families. Contact the nearest welfare office or the Department of Health and Human Services.

U.S. DEPARTMENT OF HEALTH AND HUMAN SERVICES

Administration for Children
   and Families
370 L'Enfant Promenade SW
Washington, DC 20447
202–401–9351

Type of organization: government
Public served: individuals/families,
   intermediate parties
Offers: financial assistance
Disability/chronic illness: all

Comments: Low-Income Home Energy Assistance. States disburse the funds to households with incomes that do not exceed either 150% of the poverty level or 60% of the state median income, whichever is greater. Also households with recipients of Aid to Families with Dependent Children, Social Security insurance, food stamps or certain income-tested veterans' benefits. Contact the local United Way, information and referral office, or welfare office.

U.S. DEPARTMENT OF HEALTH AND HUMAN SERVICES

Administration for Children
and Families
Washington, DC 20201
202–690–5962

Type of organization: government
Public served: individuals/families,
intermediate parties
Offers: independent living
assistance
Disability/chronic illness: developmental disabilities

Comments: States receive basic support and advocacy grants that help them enable persons with developmental disabilities to become independent, productive, and integrated into their communities. Contact regional office of Department of Health and Human Services for eligibility requirements.

U.S. DEPARTMENT OF HEALTH AND HUMAN SERVICES

Health Care Financing
Administration
East High Rise Bldg., Rm. 200
6325 Security Blvd.
Baltimore, MD 21207
410–966–3870

Type of organization: government
Public served: individuals/families,
intermediate parties
Offers: medical services, financial
assistance
Disability/chronic illness: all

Comments: Medicaid provides financial assistance to the states to make payments for medical assistance on behalf of cash-assistance recipients, children, pregnant women, the aged who meet income and resource requirements, and other categorically eligible groups. For eligible services, contact local Health and Human Services office.

U.S. DEPARTMENT OF HEALTH AND HUMAN SERVICES

Health Care Financing
Administration
Meadows East Bldg., Rm. 300
Baltimore, MD 21207
410–965–8050

Type of organization: government
Public served: individuals/families
Offers: medical services
Disability/chronic illness: those conditions that have been recognized by the Social Security Administration as disabling to the individual

Comments: Medicare (hospital insurance) available for those over age 65 and those under age 65 who have received Social Security disability checks for 24 months or railroad retirement disability benefits for 29 consecutive months, and those who have chronic kidney disease and require kidney dialysis or transplant. Supplementary medical insurance is available for a monthly premium. Call the local Social Security office.

U.S. DEPARTMENT OF HEALTH AND HUMAN SERVICES

National Institutes of Health
  Public Information Division
Rm. 305
Bethesda, MD 20892
301–496–4143

Type of organization: government
Public served: individuals/families, general public, media, medical personnel, nonmedical professionals, researchers
Offers: information, reference material, publication(s), research material
Disability/chronic illness: all

Comments: Contact the Public Information Division for information on heart and vascular system, lungs, blood, arthritis, musculoskeletal and skin diseases, diabetes, endocrinology and metabolism, digestive diseases and nutrition, kidney diseases, urology and hemotology, neurological disorders, allergy, immunology and transplantation, genetics, cellular and molecular basis of disease and vision.

U.S. DEPARTMENT OF HEALTH AND HUMAN SERVICES

President's Committee on
  Mental Retardation
Washington, DC 20201
202–619–0634

Type of organization: government
Public served: individuals/families, intermediate parties
Offers: information
Disability/chronic illness: mental retardation

Comments: The Committee's objectives are to advise and assist the president on all matters pertaining to mental retardation; study national, state, and local efforts; help coordinate federal activities; facilitate communication between federal, state, and local agencies; inform the public about mental retardation; and mobilize support for related activities. This primarily means making information available.

U.S. DEPARTMENT OF HEALTH AND HUMAN SERVICES

Public Health Services
Parklawn Bldg., Rm. 7C-08
5600 Fishers Ln.
Rockville, MD 20857
301–443–3706

Type of organization: government
Public served: individuals/families, intermediate parties
Offers: diagnostic services, counseling, financial assistance, rehabilitative services, housing
Disability/chronic illness: mental illness, substance abuse

Comments: Projects for Assistance in Transition from Homelessness (PATH). Objective is to provide financial assistance to states to support services for individuals who are suffering from serious mental illness and substance abuse, and are homeless or at imminent risk of becoming homeless. Contact the local United Way or the information and referral office to locate the local agency and inquire about available services.

U.S. DEPARTMENT OF HEALTH AND HUMAN SERVICES
Public Health Services
Parklawn Bldg., Rm. 9–12
5600 Fishers Ln.
Rockville, MD 20857
301–443–9371

Type of organization: government
Public served: individuals/families, general public, medical personnel, nonmedical professionals, researchers, intermediate parties

Offers: information, diagnostic services, publication(s), medical services, research material
Disability/chronic illness: Alzheimer's disease and related disorders

Comments: Demonstration grants given to states to assist them in carrying out demonstration projects for planning, establishing, and operating programs for program development, service delivery, and dissemination of information. Although this program is for demonstration projects, individuals with Alzheimer's disease and their families may obtain some services. Contact the Washington office for a program near you.

U.S. DEPARTMENT OF HEALTH AND HUMAN SERVICES
Public Health Services
Parklawn Bldg., Rm. 9A-05
Rockville, MD 20857
301–443–6745

Type of organization: government
Public served: individuals/families, medical personnel, nonmedical professionals, intermediate parties
Offers: financial assistance
Disability/chronic illness: HIV (Human Immunodeficiency Virus), AIDS

Comments: HIV Emergency Relief Project Grants go to metropolitan areas hit hard with AIDS. Funds go to public or private nonprofit entities that provide for the development, organization, coordination, and operation of more effective and cost-efficient systems for the delivery of essential services. Several programs provide grants for the delivery of these services. Call local Health/Human Services offices for these programs.

U.S. DEPARTMENT OF HEALTH AND HUMAN SERVICES

Public Health Services
Substance Abuse and Mental
   Health Services Administration
Parklawn Bldg., Rm. 11C-22
5600 Fishers Ln.
Rockville, MD 20857
301–443–4456
FAX: 301–443–4456

Type of organization: government
Public served: individuals/families, intermediate parties
Offers: civil rights assistance/ advocacy
Disability/chronic illness: mental illness, substance abuse

Comments: Provides protection and advocacy for individuals with mental illness who are inpatients or residents in facilities rendering care or treatment and for 90 days following discharge. Also for those being admitted to or being transported to such a facility. Persons who are involuntarily confined in a municipal detention facility for reasons other than conviction of a criminal offense also receive help.

U.S. DEPARTMENT OF HEALTH AND HUMAN SERVICES

Social Security Administration
Annex, Rm. 4100
Baltimore, MD 21235
410–965–2736

Type of organization: government
Public served: individuals/families
Offers: financial assistance
Disability/chronic illness: visual impairments or other disabilities

Comments: Supplemental Security Income seeks to assure a minimum level of income to persons who have attained age 65 or are blind or disabled, whose income and resources are below specified levels. Contact local Social Security office.

U.S. DEPARTMENT OF HEALTH AND HUMAN SERVICES

Social Security Administration
6401 Security Blvd.
Baltimore, MD 21235
410–965–2736

Type of organization: government
Public served: individuals/families
Offers: financial assistance
Disability/chronic illness: black lung disease (pneumoconiosis) or other chronic lung disease arising from coal-mine employment

Comments: Disability payments for disabled coal miners and their dependents, or survivors. Contact local Social Security office.

U.S. DEPARTMENT OF HEALTH AND HUMAN SERVICES

Social Security Administration
Office of Public Inquiries
Annex, Rm. 4100
Baltimore, MD 21235
410–965–2736

Type of organization: government
Public served: individuals/families, intermediate parties
Offers: financial assistance
Disability/chronic illness: conditions determined by the Social Security Administration to be disabling

Comments: Offers disability insurance designed to replace part of the earnings lost because of a physical or mental impairment severe enough to prevent a person from working. Benefits are monthly cash payments based on past earnings of the individual. Payments are made to the individual and eligible dependents. Contact local Social Security office.

U.S. DEPARTMENT OF HOUSING AND URBAN DEVELOPMENT

Assistant Secretary for Public and Indian Housing
Washington, DC 20410
202–708–0950

Type of organization: government
Public served: individuals/families, intermediate parties
Offers: housing
Disability/chronic illness: all

Comments: To provide and operate cost-effective, decent, safe, and sanitary dwellings for lower income families through an authorized local public housing agency or Indian housing authority. Those benefiting are lower income families, including individuals who are 62 years old or older, disabled, handicapped, or the remaining member of a tenant family. Contact nearest HUD field office.

U.S. DEPARTMENT OF HOUSING AND URBAN DEVELOPMENT

Assistant Secretary for Public
    and Indian Housing
Washington, DC 20410
202–755–0950

Type of organization: government
Public served: individuals/families,
    intermediate parties
Offers: financial assistance,
    housing
Disability/chronic illness: all

Comments: Low-income housing.
Homeownership opportunities for
low-income families. Contact the
nearest HUD field office for pub-
lic housing, and the Office of
Indian Programs in Chicago,
Denver, Phoenix, and Seattle, or
the Indian Program Division in
Oklahoma City, or the Indian
Housing Division in Anchorage,
AK.

U.S. DEPARTMENT OF HOUSING AND URBAN DEVELOPMENT

Director, Title I
    Insurance Division
Washington, DC 20410
1–800–733–4663
202–708–2880

Type of organization: government
Public served: individuals/families,
    intermediate parties
Offers: information, financial
    assistance, housing
Disability/chronic illness: all

Comments: Guaranteed/insured
loans for the purchase of manu-
factured homes available to eligible borrowers. Contact HUD
headquarters for program information.

U.S. DEPARTMENT OF HOUSING AND URBAN DEVELOPMENT

Housing for Elderly and
    Handicapped People Division
Washington, DC 20410
202–708–2730

Type of organization: government
Public served: individuals/families,
    general public, intermediate
    parties
Offers: information, financial
    assistance, housing
Disability/chronic illness: all

Comments: Project grants go to
nonprofit corporations for construction or rehabilitation of supportive housing to benefit persons
with physical disabilities, or developmentally disabled or chroni-

cally mentally ill persons (18 years of age or older) with very low incomes. Contact nearest HUD field office for location of existing or proposed projects.

U.S. DEPARTMENT OF HOUSING AND URBAN DEVELOPMENT

Insured Family Development
    Division, Single Family
    Housing
Washington, DC 20410
202–708–2700

Type of organization: government
Public served: individuals/families,
    intermediate parties
Offers: financial assistance,
    housing
Disability/chronic illness: all

Comments: Offers home equity conversion mortgages, guaranteed/ insured loans to enable elderly homeowners to convert equity in their homes to monthly streams of income or lines of credit. Contact nearest HUD field office.

U.S. DEPARTMENT OF HOUSING AND URBAN DEVELOPMENT

Office of Affordable
    Housing Program
451 7th St. SW, Rm. 7158
Washington, DC 20410
202–708–0324

Type of organization: government
Public served: individuals/families,
    intermediate parties
Offers: financial assistance,
    housing
Disability/chronic illness: all

Comments: Hope for Homeownership of Single Family Homes (HOPE 3): Eligible beneficiaries are families or individuals with an income at or below 80% of area median, adjusted for family size, and who are also first-time homebuyers. Project grants are made to eligible intermediate parties. Contact nearest HUD field office for more information.

U.S. DEPARTMENT OF HOUSING AND URBAN DEVELOPMENT

Office of Affordable
    Housing Program
451 7th St. SW
Washington, DC 20410
202–708–2685

Type of organization: government
Public served: individuals/families,
    intermediate parties
Offers: financial assistance,
    housing
Disability/chronic illness: all

Comments: Home Investment in Affordable Housing (HOME program): Formula grants to intermediate parties to provide decent and affordable housing, including rentals. For rentals, at least 90% of HOME funds must benefit low- and very low-income families at 60% of area median income. Remaining 10% must be invested in families below 80% of area median. Assistance to homeowners must be to those below 80%. Contact nearest HUD field office.

U.S. DEPARTMENT OF HOUSING AND URBAN DEVELOPMENT

Office of Assisted Housing,
    Rental Assistance Division
Washington, DC 20410
202–755–4969

Type of organization: government
Public served: individuals/families,
    intermediate parties
Offers: financial assistance,
    housing
Disability/chronic illness: all

Comments: Moderate Rehabilitation, Lower Income Housing Assistance Program through authorized public housing agency or state, county, municipality, or other governmental entity or public body. Very low-income families (at 50% of median income for the area) or, on an exception basis, lower income single person who is elderly, disabled, handicapped, dis-

placed, or last in a tenant family. Contact local HUD field office.

U.S. DEPARTMENT OF HOUSING AND URBAN DEVELOPMENT

Office of Fair Housing and
    Equal Opportunity
451 7th St. SW
Washington, DC 20410
202–619–8045

Type of organization: government
Public served: individuals/families
Offers: civil rights assistance/
    advocacy
Disability/chronic illness: all

Comments: Any individual feeling aggrieved because of an alleged discriminatory action on the basis of race, color, national origin, handicap, or age in a Title 1 program may file a complaint with the Department of Housing and Urban Development. Contact the regional director for Fair Housing and Equal Opportunity at the nearest HUD regional office.

U.S. DEPARTMENT OF HOUSING AND URBAN DEVELOPMENT

Office of Fair Housing and
    Equal Opportunity
451 7th St. SW
Washington, DC 20410
202–708–0822

Type of organization: government
Public served: individuals/families,
intermediate parties
Offers: civil rights assistance/
advocacy
Disability/chronic illness: all

Comments: Architectural Barriers Act Enforcement, Section 502: ensures that all facilites owned, leased, or constructed by the federal government with specific design standards shall be accessible to physically handicapped persons. Any individual feeling aggrieved because of an alleged discriminatory action on the basis of handicap may file a complaint with the Department of Housing and Urban Development. (To file a complaint on the local level, contact the regional office.)

U.S. DEPARTMENT OF HOUSING AND URBAN DEVELOPMENT
Office of Fair Housing and
Equal Opportunity
451 7th St. SW
Washington, DC 20410
202–708–0836

Type of organization: government
Public served: individuals/families

Offers: civil rights assistance/
advocacy
Disability/chronic illness: all

Comments: Section 504 of the Rehabilitation Act of 1973 prohibits discrimination on the basis of handicap in federally assisted or federally conducted programs. Contact regional director of Fair Housing and Equal Opportunity in nearest HUD regional office.

U.S. DEPARTMENT OF HOUSING AND URBAN DEVELOPMENT
Office of Fair Housing and
Equal Opportunity
Washington, DC 20410
202–708–4252*

Type of organization: government
Public served: individuals/families
Offers: housing
Disability/chronic illness: all

Comments: *Toll-free number for filing complaints: 1–800–669–9777 (voice), or 1–800–927–9275 (TDD). Equal opportunity in housing for all without discrimination because of race, color, religion, sex, familial status, handicap, or national origin in the sale, rental or advertising of dwellings, etc.

U.S. DEPARTMENT OF HOUSING AND URBAN DEVELOPMENT
Office of Multifamily
  Housing Management
Washington, DC 20410
202–708–3730

Type of organization: government
Public served: individuals/families,
  intermediate parties
Offers: information, financial
  assistance, housing
Disability/chronic illness: all

Comments: Rent supplements, rental housing for lower income families. NO new projects are being approved. Qualified families may apply for admission to existing projects. Direct payments are provided to owners of such projects to enable renters to pay no more than 30% of their income for rent. Contact nearest HUD field office for location of existing projects.

U.S. DEPARTMENT OF HOUSING AND URBAN DEVELOPMENT
Office of Multifamily
  Housing Management
Washington, DC 20410
202–708–3730

Type of organization: government
Public served: individuals/families,
  intermediate parties
Offers: financial assistance,
  housing
Disability/chronic illness: all

Comments: Section 8 Housing seeks to aid very low-income families in obtaining decent, safe, and sanitary rental housing. NO new projects are planned; however, individuals, specifically the elderly, disabled, handicapped, or displaced, are eligible to seek rentals in existing Section 8 housing. Contact the nearest HUD field office for more information.

U.S. DEPARTMENT OF HOUSING AND URBAN DEVELOPMENT
Office of Resident
  Initiatives, HUD
451 7th St. SW, Rm. 6130
Washington, DC 20410
202–708–4542*

Type of organization: government
Public served: individuals/families,
  intermediate parties
Offers: financial assistance,
  housing
Disability/chronic illness: all

Comments: *For TDD call 1–800–877–8330 or 202–708–9300. Home Ownership and Opportunity for People Everywhere (HOPE 2) empowers low-income residents to become homeowners. Project grants available to intermediate parties, such as resident management corporations, cooperative associations, public agencies, etc. Contact Resident Initiative Specialist in the Housing Management Division of the nearest HUD field office.

U.S. DEPARTMENT OF HOUSING AND URBAN DEVELOPMENT

Policies and Procedures Division
Office of Insured Multifamily
   Development
Washington, DC 20410
202–708–2556

Type of organization: government
Public served: individuals/families, intermediate parties
Offers: financial assistance, housing
Disability/chronic illness: all

Comments: Mortgage insurance for construction or substantial rehabilitation of condominium projects. Any individual is eligible to purchase a condominium from the private profit-motivated develop-

ers, public bodies, or other sponsors who meet FHA requirements for mortgagors. Contact local directory for nearest HUD office.

U.S. DEPARTMENT OF HOUSING AND URBAN DEVELOPMENT

Single Family Development
   Division
Washington, DC 20410
202–708–2556

Type of organization: government
Public served: individuals/families, intermediate parties
Offers: information, financial assistance, housing
Disability/chronic illness: all

Comments: Guaranteed/insured loans for purchase, repair, rehabilitation, or construction of housing in older, declining areas. Multifamily sponsorship is also available. Contact nearest HUD field office. Goal is to aid in providing adequate housing for low- and moderate-income families.

U.S. DEPARTMENT OF HOUSING AND URBAN DEVELOPMENT

Single Family Development
   Division
Washington, DC 20410
202–708–2700

Type of organization: government
Public served: individuals/families,
intermediate parties
Offers: information, financial
assistance, housing
Disability/chronic illness: all

Comments: Guaranteed/insured
loans for homes in outlying areas,
open to all individuals/families.
Contact nearest HUD field office.

U.S. DEPARTMENT OF HOUSING AND URBAN DEVELOPMENT

Single Family Development
Division
Washington, DC 20410
202–708–2700

Type of organization: government
Public served: individuals/families,
general public, intermediate
parties
Offers: information, financial
assistance, housing
Disability/chronic illness: all

Comments: Guaranteed/insured
loans to make homeownership
possible for low- and moderate-
income families who cannot meet
normal HUD requirements. Counseling assistance is also available
for prospective homeowners.
Contact nearest HUD field office
for information on Mortgage Insurance—Special Credit Risks
(Section 237).

U.S. DEPARTMENT OF HOUSING AND URBAN DEVELOPMENT

Single Family Development
Division
Washington, DC 20410
202–708–2700

Type of organization: government
Public served: individuals/families,
intermediate parties
Offers: financial assistance,
housing
Disability/chronic illness: all

Comments: Guaranteed/insured
loans available for **low- and
moderate-income families** for
proposed or existing low-cost one-
to four-family housing or the rehabilitation of such housing. Any
family may apply, but families
displaced because of a natural di-
saster qualify for special terms.
Contact the nearest HUD field
office.

U.S. DEPARTMENT OF HOUSING AND URBAN DEVELOPMENT

Single Family Development
Division
Washington, DC 20410
202–708–2700

Type of organization: government
Public served: individuals/families,
intermediate parties
Offers: financial assistance,
housing
Disability/chronic illness: all

Comments: Guaranteed/insured loans for proposed, under construction, or existing one- to four-family houses, as well as for refinancing indebtedness on existing housing. Designated areas of limited housing opportunities and maximum mortgage amounts may be obtained from local HUD field offices. Anyone may apply.

U.S. DEPARTMENT OF HOUSING AND URBAN DEVELOPMENT
Single Family Development
Division
Washington, DC 20410
202–708–2700

Type of organization: government
Public served: individuals/families,
intermediate parties
Offers: information, financial
assistance, housing, food
Disability/chronic illness: all

Comments: Guaranteed/insured loans for homes in **urban renewal areas.** Any individual/family may apply. Contact nearest HUD field office.

U.S. DEPARTMENT OF HOUSING AND URBAN DEVELOPMENT
Special Needs Assistance
Program
451 7th St. SW
Washington, DC 20410–7000
202–708–4300
202–708–2565 (TDD)

Type of organization: government
Public served: individuals/families,
intermediate parties
Offers: financial assistance,
housing
Disability/chronic illness: AIDS

Comments: Housing Opportunities for Persons with Aids (HOPEWA): formula grants and project grants to provide counseling, information, and referral services to help individuals locate, acquire, finance, and maintain housing. Also offers short-term rent, mortgage, and utility payments and more. For low-income individuals with AIDS or related diseases and their families.

U.S. DEPARTMENT OF HOUSING AND URBAN DEVELOPMENT
Special Needs Assistance
Program
451 7th St. SW
Washington, DC 20410
202–708–4300

Type of organization: government
Public served: individuals/families, intermediate parties
Offers: financial assistance, housing
Disability/chronic illness: all

Comments: Responsible for Supplemental Assistance for Facilities to Assist the Homeless program, specifically for homeless families with children, elderly homeless, and handicapped individuals, through intermediary parties. Contact nearest HUD field office for information on area facilities.

U.S. DEPARTMENT OF HOUSING AND URBAN DEVELOPMENT
Special Needs Assistance
Program
451 7th St. SW, Rm. 7262
Washington, DC 20410
202–708–4300

Type of organization: government
Public served: individuals/families, intermediate parties
Offers: financial assistance, housing
Disability/chronic illness: all

Comments: Shelter Plus Care program: provides rental assistance in connection with other supportive services to homeless persons with disabilities (primarily those who are seriously mentally ill; who have chronic problems with alcohol, drugs, or both; or have AIDS, and their families). Contact nearest HUD field office for Shelter Plus Care information.

U.S. DEPARTMENT OF HOUSING AND URBAN DEVELOPMENT
Special Needs Assistance
Program
451 7th St. SW
Washington, DC 20410
202–708–4300

Type of organization: government
Public served: individuals/families, intermediate parties
Offers: financial assistance, housing
Disability/chronic illness: mental disabilities, physical disabilities

Comments: Has transitional Housing and Permanent Housing for Handicapped Homeless Persons program. Provides project grants and direct payments for specified uses. Homeless individuals and families with children should contact the Supportive Housing Program in the Regional Office of Community Planning and Development and the nearest HUD field office for information on any such housing in their area.

U.S. DEPARTMENT OF JUSTICE
Civil Rights Division
P.O. Box 37076
Washington, DC 20066
202–514–6255*

Type of organization: government
Public served: individuals/families
Offers: civil rights assistance/
  advocacy
Disability/chronic illness: all

Comments: *Office of Public Affairs, 202–514–2007 (voice), 202–514–4019 (TDD). Works to initiate actions for redress in cases involving deprivation of rights of institutionalized persons secured and protected by the Constitution or laws of the U.S. Also works to provide equal utilization of any public facility owned or operated by any state or subdivision without regard to race, religion, or national origin.

U.S. DEPARTMENT OF JUSTICE
Civil Rights Division
Chief, Public Access Section
P.O. Box 66738
Washington, DC 20035–6738
202–307–0663 (voice and TDD)

Type of organization: government
Public served: individuals/families
Offers: civil rights assistance/
  advocacy
Disability/chronic illness: all

Comments: Americans with Disabilities Act Technical Assistance Program: provides project grants for the Provision of Specialized Services and Dissemination of Technical Information program, which funds published materials, conferences, seminars, and training, and the provision of expert advisory services to ensure compliance with the Americans with Disabilities Act.

U.S. DEPARTMENT OF LABOR
Employment and Training
  Administration
Job Training Partnership Act
200 Constitution Ave. NW
Washington, DC 20210
202–219–5580

Type of organization: government
Public served: individuals/families,
  intermediate parties
Offers: vocational services
Disability/chronic illness: all

Comments: Formula grants to establish programs for youth and adults facing serious barriers to employment. Prepares them for participation in labor force by providing job training and other services that will result in increased employment and earnings, increased educational and occupational skills, and decreased welfare dependency. Handicapped individuals are included. Contact local United Way office or local chamber of commerce.

U.S. DEPARTMENT OF LABOR

Office of the Assistant Secretary
  for Veterans' Employment
  and Training
200 Constitution Ave. NW,
  Rm. S-1316
Washington, DC 20210
202–219–9110

Type of organization: government
Public served: individuals/families
Offers: counseling, vocational
  services
Disability/chronic illness: all

Comments: Disabled Veterans Outreach Program is meant to provide job training, placement, counseling, testing, and job referral to eligible veterans, especially disabled veterans of the Vietnam era. Contact regional or state director for Veterans' Employment and Training program information at the nearest state employment office.

U.S. DEPARTMENT OF LABOR

Office of the Assistant Secretary
  for Veterans' Employment
  and Training
200 Constitution Ave. NW,
  Rm. S-1316
Washington, DC 20210
202–219–9110

Type of organization: government
Public served: individuals/families
Offers: vocational services
Disability/chronic illness: service-
  connected disabilities

Comments: JTPA Title IV-c, Veterans Employment Program. Develops programs to meet the employment and training needs of service-connected disabled veterans, veterans of Vietnam era, and veterans recently separated from military service. Contact local state employment office or regional offices.

U.S. DEPARTMENT OF LABOR

Office of Worker's
  Compensation Programs
Employment Standards
  Administration
Division of Coal Mine Workers;
  Compensation
Washington, DC 20210
202–219–6692

Type of organization: government
Public served: individuals/families
Offers: financial assistance
Disability/chronic illness: black
  lung (coal workers'
  pneumoconiosis)

Comments: Benefits to disabled coal miners, their widows, and other surviving dependents of the deceased. Contact local Social Security Administration office or Coal Mine Workers' Compensation district office.

U.S. DEPARTMENT OF VETERANS AFFAIRS

Veterans Benefits Administration
Washington, DC 20420
1–800–827–1000*

Type of organization: government
Public served: individuals/families
Offers: financial assistance, living aids
Disability/chronic illness: all

Comments: *Rings in nearest local office. Automobiles and adaptive equipment available for certain qualified disabled veterans and members of the armed forces by means of direct payments for specified use. Contact nearest VA regional field office or patient representative at a VA medical center or outpatient clinic.

U.S. DEPARTMENT OF VETERANS AFFAIRS

Veterans Benefits Administration
Washington, DC 20420
1–800–827–1000*

Type of organization: government
Public served: individuals/families
Offers: financial assistance
Disability/chronic illness: service-connected disabilities

Comments: *Rings in nearest local office. Compensation for disabilities incurred or aggravated during military service according to the average impairment in earning capacity such disability would cause in civilian occupations. Contact nearest VA regional office. Study the Code of Federal Regulations 38, Parts 0–17, available at U.S. Government bookstores or at the Federal Depository Library.

U.S. DEPARTMENT OF VETERANS AFFAIRS

Veterans Benefits Administration
Washington, DC 20420
1–800–827–1000*

Type of organization: government
Public served: individuals/families
Offers: financial assistance, housing
Disability/chronic illness: permanent and total disabilities

Comments: *Rings in nearest local office. Direct Loans for Disabled Veterans provides certain severely disabled veterans with direct housing credit in connection with grants for specially adapted housing with special features or movable facilities made necessary by the nature of their disabilities. Contact the nearest VA regional office.

U.S. DEPARTMENT OF VETERANS AFFAIRS
Veterans Benefits Administration
Washington, DC 20420
1–800–827–1000*

Type of organization: government
Public served: individuals/families
Offers: financial assistance
Disability/chronic illness: all

Comments: *Rings in nearest local office. Pension for wartime veterans who are permanently and totally disabled for reasons other than a service-connected disability. Contact local veterans service officer, or VA regional office.

U.S. DEPARTMENT OF VETERANS AFFAIRS
Veterans Benefits Administration
Washington, DC 20420
1–800–827–1000*

Type of organization: government
Public served: individuals/families
Offers: financial assistance, housing
Disability/chronic illness: severe disabilities, paraplegia

Comments: *Rings in nearest local office. Specially Adapted Housing for Disabled Veterans (Paraplegic Housing) assists certain severely disabled veterans in acquiring suitable housing units, with spe-

cial fixtures and facilities made necessary by the nature of the veteran's disabilites (permanent and total disability). Contact nearest VA regional office.

U.S. DEPARTMENT OF VETERANS AFFAIRS
Veterans Benefits Administration
Washington, DC 20420
1–800–827–1000*

Type of organization: government
Public served: individuals/families
Offers: education, financial assistance
Disability/chronic illness: all

Comments: *Rings in nearest local office. Survivors and Dependents of Disabled Veterans educational assistance provides partial support to those seeking to advance their education who are qualifying spouses, surviving spouses, or children of deceased veterans or veterans who have a 100% service-connected disability, or are MIA (Missing in Action) or currently are prisoners of war. Restrictions apply. Contact VA regional office.

U.S. DEPARTMENT OF VETERANS AFFAIRS
Veterans Benefits Administration
Washington, DC 20420
1–800–827–1000*

Type of organization: government
Public served: individuals/families, intermediate parties
Offers: financial assistance, housing
Disability/chronic illness: all

Comments: *Rings in nearest local office. Veterans housing, guaranteed/insured loans to assist veterans, certain service personnel, and certain unremarried surviving spouses. Helps to obtain credit for the purchase, construction, or improvement of homes on more liberal terms than are generally available to nonveterans. Contact VA regional offices.

U.S. DEPARTMENT OF VETERANS AFFAIRS

Veterans Benefits Administration
Washington, DC 20420
1–800–827–1000*

Type of organization: government
Public served: individuals/families
Offers: information
Disability/chronic illness: all

Comments: *Rings in nearest local office. Veterans information and assistance provides all necessary information and assistance to potential claimants and other interested parties about veterans benefits.

U.S. DEPARTMENT OF VETERANS AFFAIRS

Veterans Benefits Administration
Washington, DC 20420
1–800–827–1000*

Type of organization: government
Public served: individuals/families
Offers: education, vocational services
Disability/chronic illness: all

Comments: *Rings in nearest local office. Vocational Rehabilitation for Disabled Veterans provides all services and assistance necessary to enable service-disabled veterans and service persons hospitalized, pending discharge, to achieve maximum independence in daily living and, to the maximum extent feasible, to become employable and to obtain and maintain suitable employment. Contact nearest VA regional office.

U.S. DEPARTMENT OF VETERANS AFFAIRS

Veterans Benefits Administration
Washington, DC 20420
1–800–827–1000*

Type of organization: government
Public served: individuals/families
Offers: education, vocational services
Disability/chronic illness: all

Comments: *Rings in nearest local office. Vocational Training for Certain Veterans Receiving VA Pension program offers direct payments, advisory services, and counseling to assist new pension recipients to resume and maintain gainful employment by providing vocational training and other services. This is a temporary program. Contact nearest VA regional office.

U.S. DEPARTMENT OF VETERANS AFFAIRS
Veterans Health Administration
Administrative Services (161B1)
Washington, DC 20420
202–535–7384

Type of organization: government, medical facility
Public served: individuals/families
Offers: medical services
Disability/chronic illness: all

Comments: VA hospitalization, and hospital-based home care. Criteria for determining eligibility for veterans to be hospitalized can be determined by contacting the nearest VA medical center or outpatient clinic patient representative. National office is room 114A and telephone is 202–535–7530 for the home care.

U.S. DEPARTMENT OF VETERANS AFFAIRS
Veterans Health Administration
Assistant Chief Medical Director for Geriatrics & Extended Care (114)
Washington, DC 20420
202–535–7179

Type of organization: government, medical facility
Public served: individuals/families
Offers: medical services, housing
Disability/chronic illness: all

Comments: VA nursing home care is available for veterans who meet certain criteria. Contact the nearest VA medical center or outpatient clinic patient representative.

U.S. DEPARTMENT OF VETERANS AFFAIRS
Veterans Health Administration
Assistant Chief Medical Director for Geriatrics & Extended Care (114A)
Washington, DC 20420
202–535–7530

Type of organization: government
Public served: individuals/families
Offers: support group(s), counseling, medical services, housing
Disability/chronic illness: all

Comments: VA Domiciliary Care provides the least intensive level of VA inpatient care for ambulatory veterans. Provides necessary inpatient medical care and physical, social, and psychological support services in a therapeutic environment. Contact nearest VA medical center or outpatient clinic patient representative for more information.

U.S. DEPARTMENT OF VETERANS AFFAIRS

Veterans Health Administration
Assistant Chief Medical Director
 for Geriatrics & Extended
 Care (114B)
Washington, DC 20420
202–535–7538

Type of organization: government
Public served: individuals/families
Offers: medical services, housing
Disability/chronic illness: all

Comments: Veterans State Domiciliary Care, State Nursing Home, or State Hospital Care is provided by the states that have State Veterans Homes. Veterans must meet certain criteria set by the VA and those set by the state in which the domiciliary or nursing home is located. For more information, contact the patient representative at the nearest VA medical center or outpatient center, or the county veterans' service office.

U.S. DEPARTMENT OF VETERANS AFFAIRS

Veterans Health Administration
Associate Deputy Chief Medical
 Director for Clinical
 Programs (117D)
Washington, DC 20420
202–535–7637

Type of organization: government
Public served: individuals/families
Offers: support group(s), counseling, medical services, rehabilitative services
Disability/chronic illness: visual impairments

Comments: Operates Blind Veterans Rehabilitation centers and clinics, which assist in the rehabilitation of blind veterans by providing personal and social adjustment programs and medical or health-related services for eligible blind veterans at selected VA medical centers maintaining blind rehabilitation centers. Contact nearest VA medical center or outpatient clinic patient representative. Most counties have a veterans service officer.

U.S. DEPARTMENT OF VETERANS AFFAIRS

Veterans Health Administration
Director Administrative Services
(161B2)
Washington, DC 20420
202–535–7384

Type of organization: government, medical facility
Public served: individuals/families
Offers: medical services
Disability/chronic illness: all

Comments: Veterans Outpatient Care program provides for medical and dental services, medicines, and medical supplies (including prosthetic appliances) to eligible veterans. To determine eligibility, contact the patient representative at the nearest VA medical center or outpatient clinic.

U.S. GENERAL SERVICES ADMINISTRATION

Consumer Information Center
Washington, DC 20405
202–501–1794

Type of organization: government
Public served: individuals/families, general public, media, intermediate parties

Offers: information, reference material, publication(s)
Disability/chronic illness: all

Comments: Works to assist federal agencies in releasing information of interest to consumers, and to increase public awareness of the availability of this information.

U.S. GENERAL SERVICES ADMINISTRATION

Federal Information Center
KLL-I
Washington, DC 20405
301–722–9098*

Type of organization: government
Public served: individuals/families, general public
Offers: information, reference material, publication(s), research material
Disability/chronic illness: all

Comments: *Check 800 directory assistance for nearest Federal Information Center. Purpose is to provide service to the public for questions about federal agencies. Callers can receive the desired information or an accurate referral to the office that can best help them.

U.S. GOVERNMENT PRINTING OFFICE
Depository Libraries for
  Government Publications
Chief, Library Division
Library Programs Service,
  Stop SL
Washington, DC 20401
202-512-0571
202-512-1114

Type of organization: government
Public served: individuals/families,
  general public, media, researchers, intermediate parties
Offers: information, reference
  material, publication(s)
Disability/chronic illness: all

Comments: Provides a class of libraries in the U.S. and its posses-
sions in which certain government
publications are deposited by the
Superintendent of Documents for
the use of the public. There are
1,405 throughout the U.S. Contact your local library for information on the closest one.

U.S. GOVERNMENT PRINTING OFFICE
Government Bookstore
710 North Capitol St. NW
Washington, DC 20401
202-512-0132
FAX: 202-512-1355

Type of organization: government
Public served: individuals/families,
  general public, media, researchers, intermediate parties
Offers: information, reference
  material, publication(s)
Disability/chronic illness: all

Comments: There are 23 government bookstores located throughout the U.S. Check with directory
assistance for the one nearest you.

U.S. LIBRARY OF CONGRESS
Books for the Blind and
  Physically Handicapped
1291 Taylor St. NW
Washington, DC 20542
202-707-5100

Type of organization: government
Public served: individuals/families,
  nonmedical professionals
Offers: information, reference
  material, publication(s)
Disability/chronic illness: visual
  impairments, physical
  disabilities

Comments: Provides library service to the blind and physically
handicapped residents of the U.S.
and its territories and to American
citizens living abroad. There are
books on cassette and disc, in
braille, and talking-book and
recorded-cassette machines. There

are 56 regional libraries and 88 subregional libraries in the U.S. Check with your local public library.

U.S. NATIONAL COUNCIL ON DISABILITY

800 Independence Ave. SW, Ste. 814
Washington, DC 20591
202–267–3846

Type of organization: government
Public served: individuals/families, intermediate parties
Offers: civil rights assistance/ advocacy
Disability/chronic illness: all

Comments: Purpose is to develop, recommend, and monitor the effectiveness of public policies for persons with disabilities and advise the president and Congress, and disseminate information to people with disabilities. Public and private nonprofit institutions, and individuals are eligible to apply for project grants.

U.S. OFFICE OF PERSONNEL MANAGEMENT

Affirmative Recruiting and Employment
1900 E St. NW
Washington, DC 20415
202–606–0870

Type of organization: government
Public served: individuals/families
Offers: vocational services
Disability/chronic illness: all

Comments: Federal Employment for Individuals with Disabilities, Selective Placement Program encourages federal agencies to provide assistance to persons with disabilities, including disabled veterans, in obtaining and retaining federal employment. Contact regional offices of Office of Personnel Management, Federal Employment Information Centers, and/or Federal Employment Information Test Centers.

U.S. OFFICE OF PERSONNEL MANAGEMENT

Staffing Policy and Operations
1900 E St. NW, Rm. 6504
Washington, DC 20415
202–606–0960

Type of organization: government
Public served: individuals/families
Offers: vocational services
Disability/chronic illness: all

Comments: Implements Federal Employment Assistance for Veterans, which provides assistance to veterans in obtaining federal employment. Various categories of veterans are given points toward their eligibility ratings in the Civil

Service exams. Contact nearest Federal Employment Information Center or Office of Personnel Management.

U.S. PRESIDENT'S COMMITTEE ON EMPLOYMENT OF PEOPLE WITH DISABILITIES
Washington, DC 20004
202–376–6200
202–376–6205 (TDD)
FAX: 202–376–6219

Type of organization: government
Public served: individuals/families, general public, media
Offers: information
Disability/chronic illness: all

Comments: Works with governors' committees on the employment of people with disabilities to promote employment opportunities for the disabled, through public awareness campaigns.

U.S. SMALL BUSINESS ADMINISTRATION
Associate Administrator for Procurement Assistant
409 3rd St. SW
Washington, DC 20416
202–205–6469

Type of organization: government
Public served: individuals/families

Offers: information, reference material
Disability/chronic illness: all

Comments: Procurement Automated Source System (PASS) provides profiles of potential small business bidders in response to the requests of government agencies and major corporations. Has computerized database. Small businesses, including those owned by minorities and women, arc eligible. Contact SBA regional office.

U.S. SMALL BUSINESS ADMINISTRATION
Business Initiatives, Education and Training
409 3rd St. SW
Washington, DC 20416
202–205–6665

Type of organization: government
Public served: individuals/families
Offers: information, publication(s), counseling, consultations/guidance, seminars/ workshops
Disability/chronic illness: all

Comments: Has Business Development Assistance to Small Business program, which helps the prospective as well as present small business person improve skills to manage and operate a business. Help includes workshops, management counseling (often from SCORE), business student participation in Small Business Institute Program, management courses, conferences and seminars, and educational materials. Contact nearest SBA district office.

U.S. SMALL BUSINESS ADMINISTRATION
Financing, Loan Policy
and Procedures
409 3rd St. SW, 8th Fl.
Washington, DC 20416
202–205–6570

Type of organization: government
Public served: individuals/families,
intermediate parties
Offers: financial assistance
Disability/chronic illness: all

Comments: Has Microloan Demonstration Program. Objective is to assist women, low-income, and minority entrepreneurs, business owners, and other individuals in qualified areas. SBA will make loans to intermediaries, which in turn make loans up to $25,000. Contact SBA, in Washington, to find such intermediaries in your area.

U.S. SMALL BUSINESS ADMINISTRATION
Loan Policy and
Procedures Branch
409 3rd St. SW
Washington, DC 20416
202–205–6570

Type of organization: government
Public served: individuals/families
Offers: information, publication(s), counseling, financial assistance
Disability/chronic illness: all

Comments: Oversees Direct Loan Program for low-income/high-unemployment areas. Provides direct loans, advisory services, and counseling for creditworthy individuals with income below basic needs, or businesses located in areas of high unemployment, or businesses in areas with a high percentage of low-income individuals. Contact nearest SBA office or SCORE (Service Core of Retired Executives) Services.

U.S. SMALL BUSINESS ADMINISTRATION
Loan Policy and
Procedures Branch
409 3rd St. SW
Washington, DC 20416
202–205–6570

Type of organization: government
Public served: individuals/families,
   intermediate parties
Offers: financial assistance
Disability/chronic illness: all

Comments: Guaranteed regular business loans available to small businesses that are unable to obtain financing in the private marketplace but can demonstrate an ability to repay loans granted. Includes small businesses being established, acquired, or owned by handicapped individuals. Loans can be used for a wide variety of purposes, including working capital. Contact nearest SBA district office.

U.S. SMALL BUSINESS ADMINISTRATION

Loan Policy and
   Procedures Branch
409 3rd St. SW
Washington, DC 20416
202–205–6570

Type of organization: government
Public served: individuals/families
Offers: financial assistance
Disability/chronic illness: all

Comments: Offers Handicapped Assistance Loans (HAL-1, HAL-2). Established to provide direct loans for nonprofit sheltered workshops and other similar organizations that produce goods and services, and to assist in the establishment, acquisition, or operation of a small business owned by handicapped individuals. Contact nearest SBA district office.

U.S. SMALL BUSINESS ADMINISTRATION

Loan Policy and
   Procedures Branch
409 3rd St. SW
Washington, DC 20416
202–205–6570

Type of organization: government
Public served: individuals/families
Offers: financial assistance
Disability/chronic illness: all

Comments: Offers Veterans Loan Program. Open to all veterans, provides direct loans to construct, expand, or convert facilities and to purchase building equipment or materials or working capital. Contact nearest SBA district office.

U.S. SMALL BUSINESS ADMINISTRATION

National SCORE Office
1825 Connecticut Ave. NW
Washington, DC 20009
202–653–6279

Type of organization: government,
   professional

Public served: individuals/families
Offers: information, reference material, publication(s), counseling, consultations/guidance, seminars/workshops
Disability/chronic illness: all

Comments: SCORE is the Service Corps of Retired Executives Association—volunteers who share their management experience to counsel and train potential and existing small business owners. Check with local telephone directory, chamber of commerce, or library for local office or representatives.

U.S. SMALL BUSINESS ADMINISTRATION
Office of AA/MSB & COD
409 3rd St. SW
Washington, DC 20416
202–205–6410

Type of organization: government
Public served: individuals/families
Offers: information, financial assistance
Disability/chronic illness: physical disabilities

Comments: Minority Business Development, Section 8(a). Program is designed primarily for minorities (those determined by the SBA to be socially and economically disadvantaged) or by an economically disadvantaged Native American tribe, an Alaskan native corporation or a native Hawaiian organization with demonstrated potential for success. However, physically disabled individuals may be eligible. Contact nearest SBA district office.

U.S. SMALL BUSINESS ADMINISTRATION
Office of Veteran Affairs
409 3rd St. SW
Washington, DC 20416
202–205–6773

Type of organization: government
Public served: individuals/families, intermediate parties
Offers: information, counseling, consultations/guidance, seminars/workshops
Disability/chronic illness: all (in veterans)

Comments: Has Veterans Entrepreneurial Training and Counseling (VET Program). Project grants available to design, develop, administer, and evaluate an entrepreneurial and procurement training and counseling program for U.S.

veterans. Veterans should contact nearest SBA field office for names of participants in the program.

U.S. SMALL BUSINESS ADMINISTRATION
Office of Women's
    Business Ownership
409 3rd St. SW
Washington, DC 20416
202–205–6673

Type of organization: government
Public served: individuals/families,
    intermediate parties
Offers: information, counseling,
    consultations/guidance,
    seminars/workshops
Disability/chronic illness: all

Comments: Offers Women's Business Ownership Assistance. Project grants that will establish demonstration projects for the benefit of small business concerns owned and controlled by women. The services and assistance provided by the projects are to include financial, management, and marketing training and counseling for start-up or established ongoing concerns. See Women's Business Ownership representative at the nearest SBA office.

VERY SPECIAL ARTS
John F. Kennedy Center for
    the Performing Arts
    Educational Office
Washington, DC 20566
1–800–933–VSA1
202–628–2800*
FAX: 202–737–0725

Type of organization: nonprofit
Public served: individuals/families,
    general public
Offers: information, reference
    material, publication(s),
    consultations/guidance,
    seminars/workshops,
    recreational opportunities
Disability/chronic illness: all

Comments: *For TDD call 202–737–0645. International coordinating agency for quality arts programs for individuals from 55 countries with disabilities. Purpose is to assure that individuals with disabilities have year-round opportunities to participate in educational programs demonstrating the value of the arts and to provide experiences to help them become active participants in mainstream society.

VIETNAM VETERANS AGENT ORANGE VICTIMS

P.O. Box 42130
Darien, CT 06820-0465
1-800-521-0198
203-323-7478

Type of organization: nonprofit
Public served: individuals/families
Offers: information, reference material, publication(s), medical referrals, nonmedical referrals, seminars/workshops, civil rights assistance/advocacy, research material
Disability/chronic illness: cancer

Comments: Assists veterans who were exposed to Agent Orange during the Vietnam War in obtaining needed services. Lobbies the government, monitors state and local herbicide use, and alternatives to herbicide brush management. Has speakers bureau. Holds seminars for incarcerated Vietnam veterans, educates the public on herbicides.

VOICE OF THE RETARDED

2800 Central Rd.
Rolling Meadows, IL 60008
703-253-6020
FAX: 703-253-6054

Type of organization: nonprofit
Public served: individuals/families,
medical personnel, nonmedical professionals
Offers: information, civil rights assistance/advocacy, research material
Disability/chronic illness: mental disabilities

Comments: Members include families and friends of mentally disabled and mental health care professionals and providers. Advocates for the general welfare of mentally disabled individuals by working to improve mental health care and services, monitoring related legislation, increasing public awareness of mental health issues, and providing resources to individuals, guardians, and families.

VOLUNTEERS OF AMERICA

3939 North Causeway, Ste. 202
Metairie, LA 70002
1-800-426-5934*
504-837-2652

Type of organization: nonprofit
Public served: individuals/families
Offers: information, support group(s), counseling, medical referrals, nonmedical referrals, financial assistance, rehabilitative services, vocational services
Disability/chronic illness: all

Comments: *Or 1–800–222–3196. Volunteers participate in many different programs to help disabled and elderly as well as others. Offers more than 400 programs in more than 200 communities.

WESTERN CENTER FOR MICROCOMPUTERS IN SPECIAL EDUCATION
1259 El Camino Real, Ste. 275
Menlo Park, CA 94025
415–326–6997

Type of organization: nonprofit
Public served: individuals/families, general public, nonmedical professionals
Offers: information, products
Disability/chronic illness: all

Comments: Publishes the newsletter *The Catalyst,* which includes information on computer hardware, software, and applications that are designed for special education. Voice mail reached at 415–855–8064.

WHEELCHAIR MOTORCYLCE ASSOCIATION
101 Torrey St.
Brockton, MA 02401
508–583–8614

Type of organization: nonprofit
Public served: individuals/families

Offers: recreational opportunities
Disability/chronic illness: physical disabilities

Comments: Members include handicapped persons confined to wheelchairs, interested in rediscovering the outdoors. Also institutional and individual supporters. Researches, develops, and tests off-road vehicles for quadriplegics and other severely handicapped persons. Has produced an audio-visual program showing the use of cycles by the handicapped. Provides consultation and literature-searching services.

WORLD INSTITUTE ON DISABILITY
510 16th St.
Oakland, CA 94612
510–763–4100
FAX: 510–763–4109

Type of organization: nonprofit
Public served: individuals/families, general public, media, medical personnel, nonmedical professionals
Offers: information, reference material, publication(s), consultations/guidance, civil rights assistance/advocacy, research material
Disability/chronic illness: all

Comments: Nonmembership coalition of disabled individuals with personal and professional knowledge of disability-related issues. Serves as a public policy institute seeking solutions to problems facing people of all ages who are disabled. Advocates and conducts research on personal assistance services for people with disabilities. Operates the Research and Training Center on Policy in Independent Living.

WORTON DYSLEXIA SOCIETY
Chester Bldg., Ste. 382
8600 LaSalle Rd.
Baltimore, MD 21286
1–800–222–3123 (in U.S.,
　except MD)
410–296–0232
FAX: 410–321–5069

Type of organization: nonprofit
Public served: individuals/families,
　general public, media
Offers: information, publication(s), nonmedical referrals,
　seminars/workshops
Disability/chronic illness: dyslexia,
　learning disabilities

Comments: Has 44 chapters, including ones in Canada and Israel.

YOUTH EMOTIONS ANONYMOUS
c/o Martha Bush
P.O. Box 4245
St. Paul, MN 55104
612–647–9712
FAX: 612–647–1593

Type of organization: nonprofit
Public served: individuals/families
Offers: publication(s), support
　group(s)
Disability/chronic illness: mental
　illness

Comments: Has 50 local groups. Program of Emotions Anonymous. For individuals ages 13–18 who wish to become healthier emotionally. Functions as a support group for individuals wishing to develop positive attitudes and habits. Uses the Twelve-Step Method of Alcoholics Anonymous World Services, adapted to emotional problems. Provides telephone referrals, directory, and mailing list. Maintains speakers bureau.

Disability and Chronic Illness Index

ALL, IN ADOLESCENT GIRLS

ALL, IN CHILDREN AND/OR YOUTH

ALLERGIES

ALZHEIMER'S DISEASE

AMPUTEES

AMYOTROPHIC LATERAL SCLEROSIS (Lou Gehrig's Disease)

170

TAY-SACHS
National Tay-Sachs and Allied Diseases
   Association 85

TOURETTE SYNDROME
Tourette Syndrome Association 103

VISUAL IMPAIRMENTS
See BLIND/VISUAL IMPAIRMENTS

WILSON'S DISEASE
Foundation for the Study of Wilson's
   Disease 47